Community Occupational Therapy Education and Practice

Community Occupational Therapy Education and Practice has been co-published simultaneously as *Occupational Therapy in Health Care*, Volume 13, Numbers 3/4 2001.

Community Occupational Therapy Education and Practice

Beth P. Velde, PhD, OTR/L
Peggy Prince Wittman, EdD, OTR/L, FAOTA
Editors

Community Occupational Therapy Education and Practice has been co-published simultaneously as *Occupational Therapy in Health Care*, Volume 13, Numbers 3/4 2001.

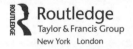

Routledge
Taylor & Francis Group
New York   London

Community Occupational Therapy Education and Practice has been co-published simultaneously as *Occupational Therapy in Health Care*™ , Volume 13, Numbers 3/4 2001.

First published by:

The Haworth Press, Inc., 10 Alice Street, Binghamton, NY 13904-1580

This edition published 2012 by Routledge:

Routledge
Taylor & Francis Group
711 Third Avenue
New York, NY 10017

Routledge
Taylor & Francis Group
2 Park Square, Milton Park
Abingdon, Oxon OX14 4RN

Cover design by Thomas J. Mayshock Jr.

Library of Congress Cataloging-in-Publication Data

Community occupational therapy education and practice / Beth P. Velde, Peggy Prince Wittman, editors.
     p. cm.
    "Co-published simultaneously as Occupational therapy in health care, vol. 13, no. 3/4, 2001."
    Includes bibliographical references and index.
    ISBN 0-7890-1405-X (alk. paper) – ISBN 0-7890-1406-8 (alk. paper)
    1. Community health services. 2. Occupational therapy. I. Velde, Beth P. II. Wittman, Peggy Prince. III. Occupational therapy in health care.

RA427 .C6184 2001
615.8′515–dc21

2001039831

Community Occupational Therapy Education and Practice

CONTENTS

ABOUT THE EDITORS

Beth P. Velde, PhD, OTR/L, is Associate Professor and Graduate Co-ordinator in the Department of Occupational Therapy at East Carolina University in Greenville, North Carolina. She holds a baccalaureate degree in zoology, master's degrees in recreation/park administration and occupational therapy, and a doctorate in educational psychology. Dr. Velde is involved in teaching both undergraduate and graduate courses. With 28 years of post-secondary teaching and research experience in diverse areas, Dr. Velde's current interests include research in the relationship between occupation and quality of life. Together with Dr. Wittman, she maintains a community-based practice in rural North Carolina where, with OT students, they provide home based occupational therapy and study the development of cultural competence, critical thinking, and interdisciplinary roles.

Peggy Prince Wittman, EdD, OTR/L, FAOTA, is Associate Professor at East Carolina University in Greenville, North Carolina. She currently teaches in both the undergraduate and graduate programs. Her clinical expertise includes working with people who are persistently and chronically mentally ill, including older adults. For the past several years she has been involved clinically in a rural health care project as part of an interdisciplinary team providing OT and PT services to area citizens. Past and current leadership roles include serving as past President of the North Carolina Occupational Therapy Association, past member of AOTA's Task Force for the Future of Mental Health Occupational Therapy, and past member of the NBCOT Commission on Continued Competency in Occupational Therapy. Dr. Wittman's research publications and interests include student development, ethics, the use of consultation in OT practice, and the practice of OT in community settings such as homeless shelters.

Occupational Therapy in the Community: What, Why, and How

Peggy Prince Wittman, EdD, OTR/L, FAOTA
Beth P. Velde, PhD, OTR/L

SUMMARY. This paper discusses ways of defining community practice. It differentiates between the terms "community-based" and "community-built" and makes the argument that community-built occupational therapy practice is the best alternative. *[Article copies available for a fee from The Haworth Document Delivery Service: 1-800-342-9678. E-mail address: <getinfo@haworthpressinc.com> Website: <http://www. HaworthPress.com> © 2001 by The Haworth Press, Inc. All rights reserved.]*

KEYWORDS. Community-based, community-built, community practice

Do not follow where the path may lead, go instead where there is not a path and leave a trail.

–Author Unknown

"A sense of community, planned communities, community-based agencies" are terms familiar to all of us. We believe, however, that while community-based occupational therapy practice is not a new idea

Peggy Prince Wittman is Associate Professor, Department of Occupational Therapy, East Carolina University, Greenville, NC 27858 (E-mail: Wittmanm@mail.ecu.edu). Beth P. Velde is Associate Professor, Department of Occupational Therapy, East Carolina University, Greenville, NC 27858 (E-mail: Veldeb@mail.ecu.edu).

[Haworth co-indexing entry note]: "Occupational Therapy in the Community: What, Why, and How." Wittman, Peggy Prince, and Beth P. Velde. Co-published simultaneously in *Occupational Therapy in Health Care* (The Haworth Press, Inc.) Vol. 13, No. 3/4, 2001, pp. 1-5; and: *Community Occupational Therapy Education and Practice* (eds: Beth P. Velde, and Peggy Prince Wittman) The Haworth Press, Inc., 2001, pp. 1-5. Single or multiple copies of this article are available for a fee from The Haworth Document Delivery Service [1-800-342-9678, 9:00 a.m. - 5:00 p.m. (EST). E-mail address: getinfo@haworthpressinc.com].

(indeed, many of us were educated about and practiced in the community 25-30 years ago), there is still a paucity of literature, research and knowledge about effective models for doing community-based education and practice. This special volume is being published to describe the efforts of some of those who have blazed a trail into the community–a viable, exciting, dynamic place for occupational therapy.

COMMUNITY OCCUPATIONAL THERAPY PRACTICE

To be effective in establishing a role for the provision of occupational therapy services in the community, the definition of community practice must be examined. If we view the community as only a physical place, institutions such as nursing homes, schools, and hospitals that happen to be located within the physical boundaries of a given community can easily be referred to as "community-based." This description views community as a "fairly boundaried social or demographic unit involving a neighborhood or people who share a common issue or interest" (Walter, 1997, p. 67). In line with this definition, the community can also be perceived as a "person's natural environment, that is, where the person works, plays and performs other daily activities" (Brownson, 1998, p. 60).

Yet community can mean more than a physical place. As Walter further states:

> I refer to community as multidimensional to describe the way in which the various dimensions that characterize community–such as people and organizations, consciousness, actions, and context–are integrally related with one another, forming the whole that is community. To develop an understanding of community, then, we need to articulate, visualize, and examine the unique qualities exhibited by each of these dimensions and how these dimensions come together to make up the complex and dynamic 'system' of community. (p. 70)

Another way of viewing community practices addresses the perspective from which services are offered. When clients, whether individuals or populations, are treated as patients who have little control over the services they receive, and occupational therapists are seen as the experts and hence the decision-makers, the perspective is simply transferring the medical model to the community. Literature in community-building

(Minkler, 1997; Walter, 1997) suggests an alternative approach. The authors of this manuscript use the following definitions to clarify their perspective (G. Herzberg, personal communication, June 27, 2000).

Community-based practice refers to skilled services delivered by health practitioners using an interactive model with clients. This model emphasizes the strengths of a specific profession in eliminating or remediating the problems of the client. Typically, this type of practice is medical system initiated, relies on referrals from other professionals, and is on-going over time.

Community-built practice is defined when skilled services are delivered by health practitioners using a collaborative and interactive model with clients. This model emphasizes the strengths of the client and is wellness oriented. Typically such a practice eliminates or resolves client issues by providing expert knowledge that is not otherwise available to the client, is issue based, and ends when the client-defined community has effectively built the capacity for empowerment.

Thus, differences between community-based and community-built models reside in the theory bases, strategies and skills needed to be effective, and the outcomes of participation in services. Community-built practice grounds itself in health promotion and wellness theory and draws from literature in health education, urban planning, and public health. It addresses the person, the community, and environmental factors interacting to support occupational engagement. Strategies used to meet goals include needs and strength assessments for populations as well as individuals, consensus about development and implementation of programs, and collaboration in the identification of outcomes. Excellent communication and negotiation skills are needed and cultural competency is vital. Services may focus on the development of the community to support the occupational functioning of its members or toward facilitating the strengths, needs and desires of an individual regarding occupational performance. Finally, outcomes may be measured by quantitative means, qualitative methods, or simply being told by the community that services are no longer needed!

So while we recognize that occupational therapists may use the terms community-based and community-built interchangeably, our purpose in editing this collection is to provide examples of models of practice, assessment tools, and programs that are more oriented to the community-built definition. The articles in this volume illustrate occupational therapy as a collaborative initiative where those who need them guide the provision of services. A goal in most has been to empower, and to put ourselves as therapists "out of business," as community members, populations, or organizations assume their own authority, expertise, and identity.

We believe that in order to prepare occupational therapists to do community-built practice, we must educate students differently. Therefore, in this collection, Fidler challenges educators to develop curricula that address the skills and abilities occupational therapists need to fulfill roles required. Perrin and Wittman describe a demonstration project being used at one university occupational therapy program to do this, and Velde and Wittman describe a community-built project which helps students and faculty develop clinical skills with a focus on cultural competence.

Pizzi and Neufeld and Kniermann write about their use of health promotion and wellness theory and strategies in their articles. Consultation skills are used in many of the programs described in this volume; Haradon directly addresses their use in helping families to successfully adapt to changes brought about by international adoptions. Examples of program development are emphasized; in their description of the use of systems theory to analyze community organizations, Elliott, O'Neil, and Velde provide a framework for analysis and program planning. Braveman writes of his work in providing vocational rehabilitation services to persons with HIV/AIDS, and Herzberg and Finlayson discuss how they have established occupational therapy services for individuals who are homeless. And finally, while the outcomes of community-built services are varied, there appears to be agreement that quality of life is a desired outcome. Velde provides a conceptual overview of global quality of life theory as it relates to occupational therapy and gives suggestions for usable assessment instruments.

We hope that you will enjoy reading about the trailblazing efforts of your peers and colleagues and that this special collection will give you support and motivation to join them in their efforts to develop community-built occupational therapy services.

REFERENCES

Baum, C. & Law, M. (1998). Nationally Speaking: Community health: A responsibility, an opportunity, and a fit for occupational therapy. *American Journal of Occupational Therapy, 51*, 7-10.

Minkler, M. (Ed.) (1997). *Community organizing and community building for health.* New Brunswick, NJ: Rutgers University Press.

Walter, C.L. (1997). Community building practice. In M. Minkler (Ed.), *Community organizing and community building for health* (pp. 68-83). New Brunswick, NJ: Rutgers University Press.

Community Practice:
It's More than Geography

Gail S. Fidler, OTR/L, FAOTA

SUMMARY. Changing the arena of occupational practice to include the community requires more than physically establishing practice in a community site. Community practice will only thrive if practitioners are adequately prepared. This means post secondary educational institutions must develop curricula upon a broad base of knowledge, focus upon theory related to occupational science, and move from a teacher based to learner based educational program. *[Article copies available for a fee from The Haworth Document Delivery Service: 1-800-342-9678. E-mail address: <getinfo@haworthpressinc.com> Website: <http://www.HaworthPress.com> © 2001 by The Haworth Press, Inc. All rights reserved.]*

KEYWORDS. Post secondary education, arena of practice

The changing health care system is having a significant impact on the practice of occupational therapy. Among a number of concerns is the diminishing number of hospital-based positions. This reality is exerting pressure to move into the community or an alternative practice site. Community practice opens a wealth of opportunities for occupational therapy. In this setting lies the challenge to broaden our parameters, to clarify, apply and critique the efficacy of our testimony to holism, the quality of life and the role of occupation in the shaping of a society and a

---

Gail S. Fidler is self-employed in Pompano Beach, Florida. Address correspondence to: 630 SW 6th Street, Sough Garden Villa #SG64, Pompano Beach, FL 33060.

[Haworth co-indexing entry note]: "Community Practice: It's More than Geography." Fidler, Gail S. Co-published simultaneously in *Occupational Therapy in Health Care* (The Haworth Press, Inc.) Vol. 13, No. 3/4, 2001, pp. 7-9; and: *Community Occupational Therapy Education and Practice* (eds: Beth P. Velde, and Peggy Prince Wittman) The Haworth Press, Inc., 2001, pp. 7-9. Single or multiple copies of this article are available for a fee from The Haworth Document Delivery Service [1-800-342-9678, 9:00 a.m. - 5:00 p.m. (EST). E-mail address: getinfo@haworthpressinc.com].

daily life. The everyday life of a community, its mix of people, their needs, concerns, joys and struggles, offers an unparalleled opportunity to define our discipline, research its potential, and extend its boundaries well beyond the current limits of our medically-based practice.

However, the transition from hospital to a community-built and based practice carries with it a significant risk if we assume that our current paradigm, which guides our education and practice, is relevant to the change. Over the years we have shaped our teaching and fieldwork experience to meet the requirements of a hospital based practice. Our singular response to the demands of managed care, HMO standards, and Medicare has further narrowed and concretized our teaching and practice focus. All too frequently these pressures have pre-empted the study and development of the broad conceptual base of our foundation. The priority focus of medicine is eradication of illness and disease. Hospitals are a critical necessity for such a mission, and they exist for that very purpose. In contrast, occupational therapy's history, the writings of its leaders and scholars, gives testimony to this developing profession's principal concern for developing and sustaining the capacities, strengths, and interests of individuals, to maximize these qualities through the process of occupation in order for each individual to achieve a productive, satisfying level of self dependency and an enhanced quality of life. Clearly, the very bases of each of these missions (medicine and occupational therapy) are different–not disparate, but different. It is understandable, then, that the hospital setting or any medically focused and managed system will naturally present roadblocks to a comprehensive practice of occupational therapy.

A paradigm for responding to the varied needs, interests and welfare of a community will differ in orientation, attitudinal and knowledge base from the one that currently guides our education and practice. Changing our arena of practice or simply adding the community as a viable service opportunity will require alternations and change in our entry-level education. Recognizing and responding to this reality is essential for successfully establishing occupational therapy as a noteworthy community service. A number of the more significant changes that will need to be addressed have been outlined in *Beyond the Therapy Model: Building Our Future* (Fidler, 1999). These changes include responding to the needs and welfare of persons with disabilities, comprehension of the person-activity and group-activity congruence, broadening our perspective of occupation, and reinforcing the inclusion of sociology, culture and history as essential components of occupational therapy education.

Altering educational patterns and outcome expectations is not a simple endeavor. We tend to teach what it is we know, what embodies predictable outcomes and what is deemed essential information. In their notable study of innovation in professional education, Boyatzis, Cowen and Kolb (1995) challenge us with the assertion that educators, especially in professional education, have lost sight of learning. They contend that teaching has replaced learning; that rather than being facilitators of learning we are in the business of passing out information. The processes of learning and teaching are different because the goals of each are different. In a related context, Johnson, Johnson and Smith (1988) observed that the ubiquitous college lecture is a process whereby the notes of the professor become the notes of the students without going through the mind of either one. Freeing our students to explore, to discover, to develop a self-reliance for one's learning should indeed be a primary outcome of professional education. It is certainly critical to moving beyond the protocols for practice.

Clearly the community is a fertile environment for verifying the authenticity of our constructs regarding the significance of occupation in the daily lives of human beings and in the formation of society. Grasping this momentous opportunity and establishing occupational therapy as a viable community service is a challenge we must not disregard. We must develop the knowledge, the skills, the attitudinal repertoire that will make it possible for us to enable our students and practitioners to discover and explore the multifaceted roles of occupation in prevention and wellness, in youth and adult education, in case management, community development, citizenship and many others yet to be discovered. A community is tailor made for such learning and for demonstrating the efficacy of occupational therapy. Being prepared to begin this journey is critical.

REFERENCES

Boyatzis, R. E., Cowen, S. S. & Kolb, D. A. (1995). *Innovations in professional education*. San Francisco: Jossey Bass.

Fidler, G. (1999). Beyond the therapy model: Building our future. *American Journal of Occupational Therapy*, 54, 99-101.

Johnson, R. T., Johnson, D. W. & Smith K. A. (1988). *Cooperative learning: An active learning strategy for the college classroom*. Minneapolis, MN: University of Minnesota.

Educating for Community-Based Occupational Therapy Practice: A Demonstration Project

Kathy Perrin, PhD, OTR/L, FAOTA
Peggy Prince Wittman, EdD, OTR/L, FAOTA

SUMMARY. This paper describes a demonstration program designed by one university Occupational Therapy program to prepare graduates to work in community-based practice settings. Faculty and students are involved in a partnership with designated community agencies to learn to assess needs, plan programs, and evaluate outcomes using a variety of research methodologies. Completion of the project is tied to the completion of a required master's degree research paper. Results of the first year of the project have been largely successful and those involved look forward to continuing the project in the future. The project is described and recommendations for change based on these results are presented. *[Article copies available for a fee from The Haworth Document Delivery Service: 1-800-342-9678. E-mail address: <getinfo@haworthpressinc.com> Website: <http://www.HaworthPress.com> © 2001 by The Haworth Press, Inc. All rights reserved.]*

KEYWORDS. Community practice, education

Kathy Perrin is Chair, Division of Human Performance Sciences, University of Mary, 7500 University Drive, Bismarck, ND 58504-9652 (E-mail: kperrin@umary.edu). Peggy Prince Wittman is Associate Professor, OT Department, East Carolina University, 306 Belk Building, Greenville, NC 27858 (E-mail: wittmanm@mail.ecu.edu). Please address all correspondence to the second author.

[Haworth co-indexing entry note]: "Educating for Community-Based Occupational Therapy Practice: A Demonstration Project." Perrin, Kathy, and Peggy Prince Wittman. Co-published simultaneously in *Occupational Therapy in Health Care* (The Haworth Press, Inc.) Vol. 13, No. 3/4, 2001, pp. 11-21; and: *Community Occupational Therapy Education and Practice* (eds: Beth P. Velde, and Peggy Prince Wittman) The Haworth Press, Inc., 2001, pp. 11-21. Single or multiple copies of this article are available for a fee from The Haworth Document Delivery Service [1-800-342-9678, 9:00 a.m. - 5:00 p.m. (EST). E-mail address: getinfo@haworthpressinc.com].

11

While occupational therapy leaders have encouraged the profession to move from institutionally-based to community-based practice for the past 20 years, recent shifts in employment opportunities have made this a necessity if the profession is to survive. However, as McColl (1998) states:

> One of the main challenges to occupational therapists in contemplating a major shift to community practice is the extent to which our existing knowledge base supports a different kind of practice in a different kind of environment . . . we need to evaluate the knowledge base in occupational therapy for applicability to community practice, or organize this knowledge around issues that are pertinent to community practice, and to identify areas for knowledge development. (p. 11)

As part of the curriculum review process and the transition to an entry level master's degree program, faculty at the University of Mary Occupational Therapy Department in Bismarck, North Dakota, decided to explore ways that knowledge and skills for doing community-based practice could be taught and learned. As a result of discussions between faculty members, their program consultant, and the University administration, a commitment was made in spring 1999 to create a service learning opportunity to develop student community practice skills. This paper describes that model and discusses its initial implementation. While only the first year's activities of the project have been completed and evaluated to date, the entire project as planned is presented in this paper.

LITERATURE REVIEW

Before beginning the "Community Partners in Service Project," relevant literature was reviewed. Helpful resources were found in documents published by the Community-Campus Partnerships for Health (CCHP) including their publication *Community-Campus Partnerships for Health* (1997) that describes a variety of models being used by health educators. Occupational therapy authors familiar with practice in community-based settings provided project planners with ideas (Brownson, 1998; Klugheit, 1994; Nielson, 1993; Strong, 1998). Because the occupational therapy faculty was already convinced of the merits of using service learning experiences to facilitate student development, literature on service learning was also used as a basis for project development (Ehrlich, 1996). Finally, relevant documents published by the American Occupational Therapy Association were reviewed. These included *The Guide to Occupational Therapy Practice* (Moyers, 1999), which emphasizes home and community settings as a major site of intervention, and intervention with populations as well as individuals; the American Occupational Therapy Association's Standards for Accreditation (AOTA, 1998), and material on student supervision (Gaffney, 2000). Based on this review of published literature, the Community Partners in Service Project was designed to serve as one component of the curriculum with required participation by all occupational therapy faculty and students.

Planners felt that involvement in this project would facilitate development of knowledge regarding community-based practice. In order to also incorporate the acquisition of knowledge and skills for doing research, planners opted to incorporate the use of both qualitative and quantitative research processes in a planning, implementation, and evaluation sequence which would occur developmentally throughout the curriculum. Since additional individual research projects are required in other classes in the curriculum, it was decided that the project would be done in small groups of six students with one assigned faculty member. The Project Coordinator (Department Chair) wrote a detailed description of the project with input from faculty.

PROJECT VISION AND ASSUMPTIONS

The vision statement for the Community Partners in Service Project (CPSP) is: "The CPSP exists to foster partnerships between communities and occupational therapy students and faculty that build on each other's strengths and that develop agents of change to improve health profession education, civic responsibility, and the health of populations in our communities." Guiding assumptions include the following:

- Health has been redefined from the absence of disease to include a focus on physical, mental, and social well-being and the person's ability to function optimally in his or her environment (Baum & Law, 1998).
- As health care expands service emphasis to health promotion and prevention, it becomes essential for occupational therapists to be familiar with community resources and how they serve the needs

of people across lifespans, diversities, and the continuum of care (Brownson, 1998).
- An expanded concept of health involves a person's ability to realize goals, satisfy needs and cope or change his or her environment–a reflection of community-based occupational therapy practice (Moyer, 1999).
- Clients of occupational therapy are no longer restricted to those persons already diagnosed with a medical problem, but now include individuals at risk for a disease, illness, or injury, or those who would benefit from lifestyle redesign. A client may be a group of individuals, a program, an organization, or a community (Moyer, 1999).

PROJECT OBJECTIVES

Investigation of the local community revealed opportunities for potential partnerships with a variety of agencies/groups who were compatible in need, commitment, vision and mission. Potential community partnerships included: industry, city and county government, architecture and engineering businesses, penal institutions, adult learning centers, retirement communities, social and public service agencies and programs, day programs (child and adult), primary health care and wellness clinics, and the city's department of parks and recreation. Concurrently with this process of identification of possible partners, project objectives were written with an emphasis on compliance with accreditation standards for occupational therapy educational programs (see Table 1).

The Project Coordinator examined many community agencies in a search for those with several different on-going programs which could provide learning experiences for up to eighteen students over the course of three years. From a list of potential matches, each faculty member selected one agency/group and made initial contact to explain the purpose and objectives of the project. Five agencies were selected: The City of Bismarck, a Headstart Program, Burleigh County Social Services, United Tribes (an agency serving Native Americans), and the Community Technical College and Mandan Public Schools (to address needs of students not eligible for special education services). Contact with a sixth agency was in process at the time of the writing of this article (Ruth Meier Hospitality House [an agency serving individuals who are homeless]).

TABLE 1. Student Objectives

At the end of the project, students will be able to:

KNOWLEDGE	ATTITUDE	SKILLS/BEHAVIORS
Demonstrate a working knowledge of the structure and function of a community agency; for example, its mission, goals, funding, marketing/publicity, governance, utilization patterns, staffing, and resource management.	Develop an increased comfort level interacting with persons.	Display effective communication skills and professional behavior.
	Cultivate a spirit of service and describe the benefits of such activity as a way to support professional development while contributing to community improvement.	Use teaching-learning processes with others, including identification of needs and methods to support these needs.
Evaluate the needs of clients served by the agency as to environmental, social, cultural, and developmental contextual frameworks.	Verbalize the importance of promoting the health of individuals in the community (outside institutional settings).	Fulfill requirements for the completion of the master's paper by completing the following sequential project segments:
Generate potential roles or contributions for occupational therapy (OT) in this agency or a similar agency in another place (e.g., student's hometown or location of practice).	Demonstrate respect for the values and diversity of persons in community settings.	Program Description: (1.5, 1.7, 1.8, 9.3) Environmental Scan (1.7, 1.8, 6.1, 6.2, 6.3, 6.5)
	Demonstrate an attitude of inquiry to enhance creativity and problem solving skills, especially for proposal of new occupational therapy contributions or roles.	Needs Assessment and Instrumentation (3.5, 4.1, 4.6, 5.9, 6.4, 8.7)
Analyze the interaction of person, environment, and occupation factors on performance in the context of a community or educational setting.		Needs Assessment Adm. (5.18, 7.18, 8.4) Analysis of Needs Assessment Results (2.4, 2.7, 5.1, 5.6) Review of Literature (8.2, 8.3, 8.4, 8.5) Strategy Identification (7.8, 9.7) Plan for Strategy Implementation (5.12, 5.13, 7.9, 7.13, 7.14, 7.15) Implement Strategies (5.6, 5.8, 5.12, 5.13, 5.19) Outcome Evaluation (1.9, 5.18, 8.4, 8.7) Outcome Evaluation Research Report (7.18, 8.7, 8.8) Presentation of Results (2.4, 2.6, 7.19, 8.8, 9.3)

PROJECT OPERATIONALIZATION

Table 2 summarizes each step of the project with details provided in the text.

During semester one, students engage in service to the community with a variety of programs which they self-select. This initial experience provides students with an overview of services available to citizens in the local community and the mechanics of their operation (e.g., how one is referred or enters in as a recipient of services, processes associated with service provision, collaboration within and outside the agency, and so forth). To insure accountability throughout the entire project process, each student is required to keep a journal of each visit. All journal entries are maintained in student portfolios. A service verification record and journal entries are submitted to the assigned faculty member (preceptor) at midterm and on the last school day prior to final exam week each semester.

In a class during the last week of semester one, faculty preceptors provide a two- to three-minute overview of their designated site. Students are asked to provide their first, second, and third choices for sites and are then matched. Up to six students are matched with a community site and preceptor for the next five academic segments. Students are notified of their match at the onset of semester two. Expectations for students, faculty, and agency coordinators are explained, and a contract is signed which clarifies responsibilities. At this time, project objectives are given to students.

TABLE 2. Steps for Completion of CPSP

SEMESTER	STEP	ASSIGNMENT
1		Community site visits
2	1	Descriptive accounts, environmental scan, needs assessment plan (Fieldwork I experience)
3	2 3	Administration of needs assessment Analysis of needs assessment
4	4 5	Review of literature Identification of strategies and methods
5 - Summer Session		Completion of draft of chapters 1, 2, 3 of master's research paper; choose research methodology
6	6	Strategy Implementation (including program evaluation) Completion of draft of chapters 4, 5 of research paper
7	7	Analysis of program evaluation/outcomes data
8	8	Preparation of poster presentation Completion of final research paper

Student groups now make their initial visits to their community sites with their preceptor to meet agency personnel and clients and to acclimate to the site environment. Schedules for future visits are arranged, and students sign a contract of commitment. Following this first visit, students function in a community service role as Level I Fieldwork students to complete a variety of tasks at the request of the community site and in keeping with the mission, philosophy, and goals of the University and occupational therapy program. Simultaneously, students learn about a population and the daily occupations of the individuals who comprise that population.

Throughout semester two of community visits, students gather information through observation and interaction with the individuals in the setting in order to complete a descriptive account of their observation and an environmental scan pertinent to the setting. A formal needs assessment plan to identify components for preassessment (exploration), assessment (data gathering), and post-assessment (utilization) phases is then generated by students, agency representatives, and the faculty preceptor.

During semester three, students are required to submit their needs assessment plan proposal and a copy of their instrumentation to the University Institutional Review Board and upon approval, administer their needs assessment, and analyze the results of the needs assessment. Faculty and students attend a Community Partners in Service seminar at the beginning of the semester to learn about instrumentation, focus groups, and other data gathering methods. Students and their preceptors partner with agency representatives to design several elements associated with the needs assessment process (e.g., content of focus group questions and questionnaires). Once needs assessment data has been collected, teams participate in a second seminar on the topic of data analysis. Results of the data analysis are shared with appropriate members of the community agency or program. Throughout the semester, students meet with their respective preceptors on a regularly scheduled basis to review materials, plans, schedules, and assignments and for reflective discussions.

During the 4th semester, students complete a review of literature relevant to their project. A seminar which highlights skills for doing a literature review is held at the onset of the semester and an additional seminar is held midterm on outcome evaluation. Both seminars are attended by student teams and their preceptors. Students and faculty meet with agency representatives to determine which programming strategy(ies) and methods will be implemented, again recognizing the mission, philosophy and goals of the agency and the University and attending to programmatic needs such as time, effort, obligation of both partners, and cost.

During the following required summer session (semester 5), students choose their research methodology, and, using knowledge gained in previous semesters, write chapters 1, 2, and 3 (as a group) of their master's degree research paper. Then, in semester 6, with support and approval of the community site and preceptor, student teams implement at least one strategy to address a prioritized need. Program evaluation data is gathered and chapters 4 and 5 of the research paper are written.

During semester 7, program evaluation data is analyzed. Additionally, in order to have an experience in role modeling and supervising Level I Fieldwork students who are beginning their Community Partners in Service Project, students meet with Year One students assigned to the community agency as part of the orientation for new community student partners.

Finally, upon return to campus following Level II Fieldwork in semester 8, students prepare a poster presentation and finalize their research papers. Individuals from the community agency who have been active participants in the Community Partners Service Project, members of the University community, and other students and guests are invited to a Poster Session Colloquium.

RESULTS

While the entire plan as described above has not been implemented, feedback has been gathered from students, faculty, and agency personnel using an open-ended questionnaire and student journal entries following the first year of project implementation. This anecdotal data about completion of descriptive accounts, the environmental scan, and the needs assessment plan shows that participants are largely positive about their first year activities. Elements of the project which were most liked by students included the opportunity to work with clients early in their academic program, the opportunity to work closely with their designated faculty preceptor, and learning more about different cultures.

Constructive feedback from students centered on the difficulty of scheduling agency visits with their peers, agency personnel, and faculty. Students also requested more "structure" and clarity of project expectations in the beginning, and some felt that they needed more attention from their faculty mentor. There was mixed feedback about the requirement to work in peer groups; while many students enjoyed the opportunity to get to know their peers better, they also commented on the difficulty of working in groups. Finally, students consistently asked for more credit hours for the amount of work they did on their projects.

Faculty remain enthusiastic about the project but they suggested that expectations for successful completion of each step of the project be clarified to all involved parties. They enjoyed working with their assigned community agency but stated that coordinating schedules was difficult. Agency personnel are extremely positive about the results of the first year's activities and comment that they are anxious to get programs started and see first-hand what occupational therapy will do for their clients.

RECOMMENDATIONS

Based on the data obtained thus far, several recommendations for changes to the project's structure have been made. First, while this project was initially linked to course credit in a designated course every semester, it was very difficult to assure that course content matched the needs for knowledge and skills required for completion of project components. Thus, a series of courses titled "Community Partners in Service Seminar" was created to occur in successive semesters beginning with semester 2. Each seminar course is one credit hour and provides back ground information necessary for project assignment completion. Preceptor and student sessions are included in these seminars to provide a forum for discussion, reflection, and performance evaluation. Community service hours (10 per semester) accumulate into a Fieldwork I experience supervised by the designated project faculty member. At the conclusion of the CPSP students have a minimum of 50 hours of Level I Fieldwork experience that results in one credit. Even with this adjustment, however, faculty remain concerned about the potential conflict between curriculum requirements to do community service for which there is no credit attached, but for which students must pay tuition. Because it is difficult to assure that the appropriate knowledge and skills needed for doing the project successfully are concurrently taught in classes, faculty must be prepared to provide information for doing the project assignments for their assigned student groups on an "as needed" basis. Efforts to allocate time and credit for project seminars and requirements is a continuing challenge.

Faculty involved in the CPSP project were excited and enthusiastic about it initially and have been very willing to do their part to make it successful. They have, however, identified several essential bodies of knowledge and skills for initiating and completing this project. These include the following: (1) assurance of faculty expertise in both quantitative and qualitative research methodologies; (2) adequate student preparation in terms of research knowledge and project expectations; (3) adequate community agency preparation in terms of expectations and knowledge of occupational therapy services. These needs will be met by having a four hour orientation seminar in semester 2 and a requirement that students meet with their designated faculty member for 16 hours/semester for supervision. This time will be used to review assignments, learning experiences, and provide feedback. Since individual student needs for structure always vary tremendously, faculty continue to explore how much expertise to share with students and how much independent learning to expect from students.

Some disparity between needs of agencies, students, and faculty was evident. For example, some agencies felt that they knew what occupational therapy could do and wanted programming to commence immediately without a needs assessment. In one case, students consistently had to deal with clients not attending their scheduled activities. While these problems were solved, they certainly reinforce the need for good communication between all parties.

Finally, while students kept their required journals, they were difficult to compare due to variation in style and content. Faculty is considering using some structure. For example, the use of standardized sentence stems may help students learn the art and importance of reflecting on their experiences and provide faculty with a more standardized way to compare responses and use qualitative research methods to analyze journal entries.

CONCLUSION

In conclusion, during its first year of operation, the Community Partners in Service Project has successfully helped students learn about the importance of doing community-based occupational therapy practice. Through a structured process of analyzing a specific community agency's mission and goal statements, program offerings, and population served, both faculty and students have developed greater appreciation for community-based programs. Additionally, students have enjoyed the service learning opportunities required by the project as a way of getting "hands-on" experiences in practice settings. They have marketed their occupational therapy skills by explaining to a variety of people what occupational therapy is and what it can offer to consumers in non-medical environments. Students, faculty, and community agency partners look forward to the second year of the project when concrete programming based on needs assessment data will be done.

REFERENCES

The American Occupational Therapy Association. (1998). *Standards for an Accredited Program in Occupational Therapy.* Bethesda, MD. The American Occupational Therapy Association.

Baum, C. & Law, M. (1998). Nationally speaking-community health: A responsibility, and opportunity, and a fit for occupational therapy. *American Journal of Occupational Therapy, 52,* 7-10.

Brownson, C.A. (1998). Funding community practice: Stage 1. *American Journal of Occupational Therapy, 52,* 60-64.

Community-Campus Partnerships for Health. (1997). *A guide for developing community-responsive models in health professions education.* UCSF Center for the Health Professions, San Francisco, CA.

Ehrlich, T. (1996). *Service-Learning in Higher Education.* San Francisco, CA. Jossey-Bass.

Gaffney, D. (2000, January 17). How does supervision change as students progress? *Occupational Therapy Practice,* 7-8.

Klugheitt, M. (1994). An appreciation for the role of occupational therapy in community mental health treatment. *Mental Health Special Interest Section Newsletter, 17(1),* pp. 1-2.

McColl, M.A. (1998). What do we need to know to practice occupational therapy in the community? *American Journal of Occupational Therapy, 52,* 11-18.

Moyer, P. (1999). The guide to occupational therapy practice. *American Journal of Occupational Therapy, 53,* 247-295.

Nielson, C. (1993). Occupational therapy and community mental health: A new and unprecedented turn. *Mental Health Special Interest Section Newsletter, 16(3),* pp. 1-2.

Strong, S. (1998). Meaningful work in supportive environments: Experiences with the recovery process. *American Journal of Occupational Therapy, 52,* 31-38.

Helping Occupational Therapy Students and Faculty Develop Cultural Competence

Beth P. Velde, PhD, OTR/L
Peggy Prince Wittman, EdD, OTR/L, FAOTA

SUMMARY. Given the need for health professionals, including occupational therapists, to be able to work with individuals and populations from a variety of cultures, this paper describes a qualitative study in which faculty and students from an occupational therapy program have been immersed in a community-built program serving African American, elderly citizens. Cultural competency and its measurement are addressed and used to assess positive results from the study. *[Article copies available for a fee from The Haworth Document Delivery Service: 1-800-342-9678. E-mail address: <getinfo@haworthpressinc.com> Website: <http://www.HaworthPress.com> © 2001 by The Haworth Press, Inc. All rights reserved.]*

KEYWORDS. Cultural sensitivity, cultural knowledge, qualitative research

---

Beth P. Velde is Associate Professor, Department of Occupational Therapy, East Carolina University, Greenville, NC 27858 (E-mail: Veldeb@mail.ecu.edu). Peggy Prince Wittman is Associate Professor, Department of Occupational Therapy, East Carolina University, Greenville, NC 27858 (E-mail: Wittmanm@mail.ecu.edu).

With grateful acknowledgement to Erin Broadhurst, Meredith Caines, Heather Lee, and Christy Lee, occupational therapy students, for their work on the Tillery Project in 1999/2000.

[Haworth co-indexing entry note]: "Helping Occupational Therapy Students and Faculty Develop Cultural Competence." Velde, Beth P., and Peggy Prince Wittman. Co-published simultaneously in *Occupational Therapy in Health Care* (The Haworth Press, Inc.) Vol. 13, No. 3/4, 2001, pp. 23-32; and: *Community Occupational Therapy Education and Practice* (eds: Beth P. Velde, and Peggy Prince Wittman) The Haworth Press, Inc., 2001, pp. 23-32. Single or multiple copies of this article are available for a fee from The Haworth Document Delivery Service [1-800-342-9678, 9:00 a.m. - 5:00 p.m. (EST). E-mail address: getinfo@haworthpressinc.com].

Over the past several decades the population of the United States has become increasingly racially and ethnically diverse. Indeed, Taylor (1998) states that "the United States is the most ethnically diverse country in the world, representing 100 racial, ethnic, and cultural groups" (p. 30). Social demographers predict that populations traditionally considered minorities will increase sufficiently so there will be no numerical majority in terms of racial or ethnic group in the United States.

Harris (2000) suggests that the education of future occupational therapy practitioners may have a direct impact on the quality of health care, particularly the treatment of those culturally different than the practitioner. However, in this education

> multiculturalism cannot be casually included in or automatically assumed to be a component of our academic programs. Instead, if we are to increase our confidence in the ability of our future practitioners to practice from a multicultural perspective, it is imperative that we seriously plan educational experiences specifically designed to achieve this goal. (p. 7)

Accreditation standards for allied health programs and university education require inclusion of material relevant to cultural differences, yet the achievement of cultural competence for both faculty and students remains a challenge. The Department of Occupational Therapy at East Carolina University chose to address the development of cultural competence using the Tillery Experience. The purpose of this paper is to describe the methodology used and to report the results of a pilot research study investigating self assessed student cultural competence.

Over the past four years the Tillery experience has provided an opportunity for occupational therapy students and faculty to be immersed in an established African American community. During this experience, participants learn to listen to the expressed needs of community members and to collaboratively determine which of those needs can be best addressed through occupational therapy intervention. Further, students and faculty use reflection and discussion to identify cultural similarities and differences.

THE TILLERY EXPERIENCE

Chicken and pastry, collard greens, and 'nanner-niller' pudding; black-eyed peas with ham hocks and cornbread; baked chicken without the skin, green beans, and birthday cake–it's Tuesday noon in Tillery, North Carolina. These are the menu choices at the Resettlement Café, the local prison, and the Open-Minded Seniors luncheon held at the community center. This small North Carolina crossroads community is described as having few young families, and the once profitable farming community has been reduced to struggling peanut and cotton farms that dot the landscape. The economic base has severely declined, and most opportunities for jobs must be explored outside the Tillery community. Tillery's 3000 citizens include 98% African Americans, 75% of whom are over the age of 65, with 90% below the federal poverty level.

Working closely with the Concerned Citizens of Tillery organization, especially its Health Committee, occupational therapy faculty and students have provided home-based evaluation and intervention services to residents. In addition, they continue to carry out a phenomenological study focused on the meaningful occupations of Tillery residents that support their independence and quality of life. Occupational historians include Mrs. C., who describes making all of her own clothing by hand, without patterns, despite a shoulder injury suffered many years ago while logging her land. Mrs. F. and Mrs. W. tell of the cooking and baking they did to raise "20 head of chillen." Mr. G., an original resettlement farmer, still raises a full garden and proudly serves watermelon to his visitors. Mrs. E. teaches about a different culture, patiently explaining why she wishes to be able to get to church to sing in the "Amen" chorus.

CULTURAL COMPETENCE AND ITS MEASUREMENT

Many definitions of cultural competence are available in the literature (Dinges, 1983; Ruben, 1989; Taylor, 1994; Wykle & Ford, 1999). This current work uses the definition provided by Cross, Bazron, Dennis, and Isaacs (1989). Cultural competence is

a set of congruent behaviors, attitudes, and policies that come together in a system, agency, or among professionals and enable that system, agency, or those professionals to work effectively in cross-cultural situations. The word 'culture' is used because it implies the integrated pattern of human behavior that includes thoughts, communications, actions, customs, beliefs, values, and institutions of racial, ethnic, religious, or social groups. The word competence is used because it implies having the capacity to function effectively. A culturally competent system of care acknowledges and incorporates–at all levels–the importance of culture, the assessment of cross-cultural relations, vigilance towards the dynamics that result from cultural differences, the expansion of cultural knowledge, and the adaptation of services to meet culturally-unique needs. (p. 13)

Cross et al. (1989) reason that cultural competence occurs on a continuum from cultural destructiveness–cultural incapacity–cultural blindness–cultural precompetence–cultural competence–to cultural proficiency. They discuss the need for both systems of care and individual practitioners to be culturally proficient and identify "five essential elements for becoming a culturally competent helping professional" (p. 32). These elements include: (1) acknowledgment of cultural differences and awareness of their effect on the helping process; (2) recognition of the influence of the helping professional's own culture on actions and thoughts; (3) understanding of the effect of differences in communication, etiquette, and problem solving on relationships; (4) an appreciation for the fact that productive cross-cultural interventions are more likely to occur when mainstream helping professionals make a conscious effort to understand the meaning of a client's behavior within his/her cultural context; and (5) recognizing how to obtain knowledge about specific cultures for use in the helping encounter.

Tripp-Reimer (1999) suggests that at each stage of the continuum specific assessment of both the student's knowledge of cultural values, beliefs and behaviors and his/her skill in working with diverse groups will assist in determining a method of progressing toward cultural competence. For example, if a person's behavior indicates cultural blindness, opportunities to gain knowledge might focus on such things as:

- encyclopedic knowledge (i.e., what does s/he know about "culture"?)
- single culture knowledge (i.e., what is his/her knowledge of rural, African American, impoverished?)
- knowledge relevant to a particular clinical area (i.e., what are those sets of cultural knowledge needed to best work in community practice?)
- knowledge related to a clinical theme (i.e., pain–how does this African American cultural group interpret pain?)

Skills might focus on culturally appropriate goal setting that is culturally congruent, brokerage skills to gain access to cultural groups, interventions that are culturally relevant, and outcome evaluations that are culturally meaningful.

Based upon data obtained during the Tillery experience, students and/or faculty may not understand there is inter and intra group variability (Wykle & Ford, 1999). This variability may occur because of situational ethnicity where individual members of a cultural group reveal information dependent upon their comfort level. Additionally, each member of an ethnic group lives at some point between the traditional culture and being acculturated into the mainstream culture. This point on the acculturation continuum changes across the person's lifespan based upon individual experience. The students and/or faculty may come in contact with community residents who vary in their placement on the acculturation continuum.

Assessment of an individual faculty member's or student's position on the continuum of cultural competence should include input from a variety of people. This includes peers, other professionals, clients, and self. While self assessment is an important part of attaining cultural competence, students and faculty who are in the cultural destructiveness, incapacity, and blindness stages of the continuum may not able to accurately assess their own competence. This is supported by the findings of Jibaja, Sebastian, Kingery and Holcomb (2000), whose work indicates that students may be "at least mildly cognizant of their personal multicultural insensitivities, but they were somewhat reluctant to call themselves 'biased' " (p. 84).

THE OCCUPATIONAL THERAPY STUDY

Statements made by several of the white, 20-year-old students who were involved in the Tillery Project in 1997-1998 provided a strong impetus for further study in the area of cultural competence (Wittman, Conner-Kerr, Templeton, & Velde, 1999). Through journal and verbal responses, the students expressed the belief that the residents with whom they were working were "just like my grandma." A review of the 1997-1998 journals indicated an interesting omission: very few comments about culture. Efforts to increase faculty and student awareness of culturally based similarities and differences and the need to move beyond cultural sensitivity led to a search for other researchers addressing cultural competence.

The literature supports the use of immersion and service learning experiences as an effective method of facilitating cultural competence.

The faculty believed any experience must include elements of honest discussion between faculty and students and with members of the Tillery community. Therefore, the 1999/2000 year was planned to include elements focused on knowledge, personal awareness, effects of cultural differences on behavior and the development of cross cultural intervention that was acceptable and effective for all parties involved.

Consequently, the year began with an on campus orientation with participation by the three faculty and eight students involved. After an overview of the history and educational goals of the Tillery project, students were placed in four interdisciplinary groups and asked to construct a community. Each group was provided with materials and objects for construction of a three dimensional prototype of an ideal community. After 30 minutes, examination of the models indicated most groups included a road system, school, hospital, shops, industry, homes, and farms/gardens. The faculty facilitated a discussion of the meaning of community and the relationships of human communities to the natural and man-made environment. This was followed by a preview of what to expect the following week during a site visit to Tillery and the concept of a crossroads community.

The next week students and faculty met with leaders from the Tillery community to share expectations and to develop a common understanding of this community. Part of the discussion included the issue of names. As community leaders pointed out, historically Black women were called by their first names, with no formal acknowledgment of a surname. Sometimes the names were not their given names, but names assigned by their White owners. Therefore, faculty and students needed to address residents by a title and surname, at least until the individual specified another manner. Other presenters discussed the need to convey respect, particularly when visiting the home of a resident. This included being aware of both verbal and body language. Students then toured the community with faculty.

The following week, students and faculty met on campus to reflect upon the community meeting. It was apparent that the discussion of naming caused discomfort among participants and additional time was spent discussing the importance of names and language. Faculty also shared with students faculty concerns about evidence of "cultural blindness" from journals of previous students, and facilitated an open discussion about the value of the differences that exist among cultures. Students identified misconceptions they held regarding the Tillery community. For example, as a crossroads community Tillery has a new fire station, a small general store, a post office, and a gas station. Approximately two miles away and not visible from the main road is the community center and health clinic. Numerous churches dot the landscape. The café is further away, on a different road. This was significantly different from the students' perception (illustrated the previous week in the community building task) that communities had clearly defined, man-made boundaries. Tillery is loosely defined by geographical and man-made structures, but held together by a strong sense of history, social interaction, and political activism. This was an important outcome of the group's reflections.

Students and faculty were now ready to begin the intervention phase of the Tillery experience. Interdisciplinary occupational and physical therapy assessments and interventions with clients referred by the health coordinator were conducted in both the community center and the client's home. To better understand cultural knowledge, cultural similarities and differences, and to reflect upon cross-cultural, interdisciplinary intervention, each student kept a journal. In weekly entries the students and faculty were asked to respond to instructions written by faculty members. Examples of entry instructions included: " Close your eyes and replay your experience in Tillery. Retrace the sequence; recall your significant thoughts, feelings, team and participant interactions, objects, culture, and physical environment. Draw or write about the highlights of this experience. Reflect upon the highlights you recorded and report your observations," and "Haiku is a form of poetry through which you express yourself and your impressions of the world. Begin by naming the intervention experience you had today. Now, describe it. Name the setting, describe the setting. Then describe the feelings you have about the image. Now, go back through what you've written and underline the key words and phrases that really describe the essence of the experience. Move these around and play with them in your mind until there are only 17 syllables: one line of five syllables, one of seven syllables, and another line of five syllables."

At the end of this phase the four occupational therapy students reflected upon their experience and each identified her development regarding the cultural competence continuum. Each of the four students identified the stage of cultural blindness/cultural precompetence as the relevant position on the continuum. This was supported by written comments including: "I recognize a difference but I don't necessarily understand/value all the reasons behind their culture," and "I feel that the Tillery people would prefer us to see our differences and respect them for those differences rather than act as if we are the same." Additionally, they stated that they were looking forward to the in-depth interviews with residents who would enhance their understanding of the impact of culture on choice of occupations, interpersonal relationships, and lifestyle. The two faculty members identified themselves between the stages of cultural precompetence and cultural competence. This was supported by comments such as "I respect and value the differences I see between Tillery residents and myself," and "It's hard to understand how the history of the African American citizen and the physical attributes of Blacks continue to negatively impact this group say in comparison to poor whites."

DISCUSSION

Several challenges emerged as a result of efforts to enhance the cultural competence of faculty and students using the Tillery experience. First, it is clear that in order to facilitate movement toward competency, faculty members who supervise students must be willing to examine their own values and attitudes, to learn, to openly communicate, and to change their own behavior as needed. For example, the discussion about names was helpful to faculty as well as students; faculty now address Tillery residents using a title and their surname unless it is clear to students that residents have asked faculty to address them by their first name. Another behavioral change that faculty model involves seating during meetings with Tillery residents or members of Tillery committees. Faculty intentionally sit interspersed with Tillery members as opposed to sitting as a unit. Without reflection, discussion between faculty and Tillery residents, and feedback from students, faculty would be less able to model behavior they expect of students.

Cultural competence needs to be assessed in a variety of ways and with input from a variety of people. During this pilot study self-assessment has been important, but in the future additional methods to assess level of competence are being explored. These may include an assessment done by community residents, the Tillery Health Coordinator, peers, measurement tools identified in the literature, and/or an objective instrument developed by the authors based on the behaviors identified in the literature. Further, a pretest needs to be administered so that faculty can appropriately plan orientation, intervention, and research experiences to meet the needs of students and faculty involved. A posttest could then measure any changes on the continuum placement.

Finally, the authors continue to be interested in those variables, experiences, and teaching strategies that will facilitate or inhibit the development of cultural competence. The Tillery experience provides a relatively brief encounter with individuals from another culture; students physically spent 8-10 hours of time interacting with clients, 2-3 hours with community leaders, and 10-15 hours with each other. If more time were available for interaction with community members and leaders, would students and faculty move further toward cultural competence? Exploration of the impact of environmental factors such as meeting with residents exclusively in their homes versus also using the community center would help in teasing out the environment's effect on the development of cultural competence. The investigation of previous experiences of students and faculty, in and out of the classroom, could determine the carry over effect of personal history on cultural competence. Finally, the faculty involved question if attainment of cultural competence with one cultural group also indicates competence with all cultural groups. Investigation of the factors that generalize across cultures could assist in answering this question.

CONCLUSION

It has been a rewarding and challenging experience to work collaboratively with students in a community-built practice environment. This environment, because of its strong African American history and heritage, requires faculty and students alike to become more culturally competent in order to be effective. As Cross et al. (1989) state, cultural competence is not developed overnight but "is a developmental process for the individual and the system. It is not something that happens because one reads a book, or attends a workshop, or happens to be a member of a minority group" (p. 21). It does occur as a process integrally linked with lifelong learning and a commitment to be an effective helping professional in an increasingly diverse global world.

REFERENCES

Cross, T. L., Bazron, B. J., Dennis, K. W., & Isaacs, M. R. (1989). *Towards a culturally competent system of care* (Vol. 1). Washington, DC: National Technical Assistance Center for Children's Mental Health.

Dinges, N. (1983). Intercultural competence. In D. Landis & R. W. Brislin (Eds.), *Handbook of intercultural training* (Vol. I, pp. 176-202). New York: Pergamon Press.

Harris, C. H. (2000, March 13). Educating toward multiculturalism. *OT Practice*, 7-8.

Jibaja, M. L., Sebastian, R., Kingery, P. & Holcomb, J. D. (2000). The multicultural sensitivity of physician assistant students. *Journal of Allied Health, 29*, 79-85.

Ruben, B. D. (1989). The study of cross-cultural competence: Traditions and contemporary issues. *International Journal of Intercultural Relations, 13*, 229-240.

Taylor, (1998). Check your cultural competence. *Nursing Management, 29*, 30-32.

Taylor, E. W. (1994). Intercultural competency: A transformative learning process. *Adult Education Quarterly, 44* (3), 154-174.

Tripp-Reimer, T. (1999). Culturally competent care. In M. Wykle & A. Ford (Eds.), *Serving minority elders in the 21st century* (pp. 235-247). New York: Springer.

Wittman, P., Conner-Kerr, T., Templeton, M. S. & Velde, B. (1999). The Tillery Project: An experience in an interdisciplinary, rural health care service setting. *Physical & Occupational Therapy in Geriatrics, 17*, 17-28.

Wykle, M. & Ford, A. (Eds.). (1999). *Serving minority elders in the 21st century*. New York: Springer.

Professional Expertise of Community-Based Occupational Therapists

Lori Lemorie, OTS
Stanley Paul, PhD, OT

SUMMARY. As the health care system changes, it is increasingly important to define the roles and contributions of individual professions. The goal of this study was to identify job roles, job skills, and professional expertise of community-based therapists. The Community Practice Project survey was mailed to 200 AOTA registered community-based therapists. There were 84 (42%) surveys returned. The results provided a profile of community-based therapists. Principal roles, job skills, and areas of professional expertise were identified. Educational preparation was assessed. Respondents reported that they were not prepared to use the skills of networking, consulting, and communication. They were not prepared in expertise areas such as community resources, self-directed learning, and client-centered approach to practice. Overall, therapists expressed satisfaction with work in community-based positions. *[Article copies available for a fee from The Haworth Document Delivery Service: 1-800-342-9678. E-mail address: <getinfo@haworthpressinc.com> Website: <http://www.HaworthPress.com> © 2001 by The Haworth Press, Inc. All rights reserved.]*

At the time this study was conducted Lori Lemorie was a Master's student at Western Michigan University's Occupational Therapy Department. Address correspondence to: 1160 S. Bunn Road, Hillsdale, MI 49242. Stanley Paul is a faculty member at Western Michigan University's Occupational Therapy Department. Address correspondence to: Western Michigan University, Occupational Therapy Department, 1201 Oliver Street, Kalamazoo, MI 49008.

[Haworth co-indexing entry note]: "Professional Expertise of Community-Based Occupational Therapists." Lemorie, Lori, and Stanley Paul. Co-published simultaneously in *Occupational Therapy in Health Care* (The Haworth Press, Inc.) Vol. 13, No. 3/4, 2001, pp. 33-50; and: *Community Occupational Therapy Education and Practice* (eds: Beth P. Velde, and Peggy Prince Wittman) The Haworth Press, Inc., 2001, pp. 33-50. Single or multiple copies of this article are available for a fee from The Haworth Document Delivery Service [1-800-342-9678, 9:00 a.m. - 5:00 p.m. (EST). E-mail address: getinfo@haworthpressinc.com].

KEYWORDS. Community occupational therapy, roles, education, expertise

The number of occupational therapists practicing in community-based settings is increasing (Devereaux, 1991; Renwick, Cockburn, Colantonio, & Friedland, 1996; Townsend, 1988). This shift has been encouraged by trends in health promotion, disease prevention, cost-effectiveness, legislation, and political movements (Chui, 1998; Grady, 1995; Peat, 1991). Practicing in the community requires occupational therapists to acquire new skills, fill new roles, and use a client-centered approach to treatment (Adamson, Sinclair-Legge, Cusick, & Nordholm, 1994; Lysack, Stadnyk, Paterson, McLeod, & Krefting, 1995; Pimentel & Ryan, 1996). Practicing in the changing health care system requires the profession to show its effectiveness, define its scope, and communicate exactly what it can contribute to health care (Baum & Law, 1997, 1998; Bezold, 1989; Pew Health Professions Commission, 1993). These demands on therapists in the community are made more difficult by the fact that occupational therapy research has focused on institutional settings (McColl, 1998; Peat, 1991).

Lysack et al. (1995) published the findings of a study that identified the expertise of occupational therapists in the community. The Community Practice Project (CPP) studied physical and occupational therapists in community-based practice in the province of Ontario. The results provided a profile of the knowledge and skills needed to work in the community. In addition, principal roles, specific job skills, areas of professional expertise and educational preparation were identified. Renwick et al. (1996) used the information gathered by Lysack et al. to identify the content needed in occupational therapy curricula. Renwick et al. utilized this data to develop a community-based course for occupational therapists. The data collected greatly expanded the understanding of what community-based occupational therapists are doing in this setting. This project was a modification of the study originally done by Lysack and her colleagues (Lysack et al., 1995).

This research endeavor was designed to satisfy specific goals. This study sought to identify job roles, job skills, and professional expertise of occupational therapists practicing in the community. This study was interested in assessing educational preparation for practice in this area. This project identified areas of continuing education recommended for practice in this setting.

LITERATURE REVIEW

There is an international trend in occupational therapy showing a shift toward community-based practice (Beech, Rudd, Tilling, & Wolfe, 1999; Strickland, 1991; Townsend, 1988). Within the profession of occupational therapy, community-based practice has existed since the 1920s. West (1967) noted a shift of occupational therapists into community-based practice. Community-based practice expanded in the '60s and '70s with home health agencies and private practice (Vanier & Hebert, 1995). Devereaux (1991) found that in the '70s and '80s community settings showed the largest increase in employment of occupational therapists. Strickland (1991), while reviewing forty years of occupational therapy practice, noted that occupational therapy practice areas have significantly shifted from being primarily institutionally based, to being primarily community-based. McColl (1998) stated that 37% of occupational therapists are practicing in the community. This shift in setting is hypothesized to be the result of an increasing emphasis on health promotion and disease prevention, a changing health care system, and increasing economic constraints (Renwick et al., 1996; Vanier & Hebert, 1995).

Community-Based Roles

The shift to community-based practice has created new roles for occupational therapists. Occupational therapists are predicted to fill the role of administrator: relocating tasks to the least trained qualified individual (Chui, 1998; Strickland, 1991; West, 1967). Occupational therapists are viewed as resources for local government, community organizations, and individuals. Therapists also serve as mentors in group settings (Dressler & MacRae, 1998). Another role for occupational therapists in the community is consultant (Hurff, Lowe, Ho, & Hoffman, 1990; Pollack & Stewart, 1998). Therapists are filling the role of enabler of function. The need to be involved in networks creates the role of collaborator for occupational therapists in the community (Finlayson & Edwards, 1995; Teague, Cipriano, & McGhee, 1990; Townsend, 1988). The role of educator is becoming more prominent in community-based occupational therapy. In addition, occupational therapists are creating community-based programs specific to the needs of individual communities (Teague et al., 1990; Townsend, 1987; Vanier & Hebert, 1995). This particular role closely resembles that of an entrepreneur. Therapists are further encouraged to adopt the role of business administrator (Devereaux, 1991; Shannon, 1985). Lastly, community-based occupational therapy practice places an emphasis upon the need of therapists to adopt the role of researcher to enhance the knowledge base behind their practice (McColl, 1998; Nelson, 1997; West, 1967).

Community-Based Skills and Expertise

The changes in the health care system as well as the novel roles and the contemporary approaches to treatment developing in community settings require that community-based occupational therapists acquire new skills. The skills identified by literature may be roughly partitioned into two categories: skills that facilitate practice in the emerging health care system, and skills that facilitate practice in the community.

A review of literature shows several skills seen as essential to occupational therapy practice within the confines of the evolving health care system. Participating in the developing health care system demands that therapists accommodate increasing accountability. Ensuring cost-effective care is also a skill required for participation in the emerging health care system (Chui, 1998; Hurff et al., 1990; Pew Health Professions Commission, 1993). Therapists need to develop the skills of practicing prevention and promoting healthy lifestyles. Another skill for therapists in this environment is to effectively involve the patients and their families in the decision-making process (Finlayson & Edwards, 1995; Pew Health Professions Commission, 1993). Therapists must also be proficient at enabling function to practice within the prevailing attitude regarding health (Madill, Townsend, & Schultz, 1985; Vanier & Hebert, 1995). These skills support the conclusion that working within the emerging health care system places many demands upon the occupational therapy profession.

Practicing occupational therapy in the community is revealed by literature as requiring novel skills. Community settings are supported, maintained, and developed by therapists who are skilled at supporting, maintaining, and developing strong networks (Hurff et al., 1990; Madill et al., 1989; Townsend, 1987). Therapists must be able to understand how community organizations structure themselves, and how they are governed. Therapists also need to develop the skill of locating resources to support their programs (McColl, 1998; Townsend, 1987). The development of community-based programs requires that occupational therapists become adept at business skills (Shannon, 1985). In addition, the skill of advocating is necessary to integrate health promotion into community settings. Consultative skills are particularly important to practice in the community (Baum & Law, 1998; Finlayson & Edwards,

1995; Hurff et al., 1990). Communication and interpersonal skills are emphasized as vital to practice in the community for effective interaction on health care teams and maintaining client involvement (Adamson et al., 1994; Shannon, 1985). The breadth of these findings supports the uniqueness of community-based practice.

The Education of Community-Based Practitioners

Community-based practice uses specialized knowledge that must be included in educational curricula (McColl, 1998; Shannon, 1985). Pimentel and Ryan (1996) listed areas that community-based occupational therapists would like emphasized in curricula: (a) the environment, (b) appropriate functional activities, and (c) dealing with challenging behavior. Occupational therapists working in the community need to be prepared to function in different organizational frameworks. In this setting, therapists also need to be able to work effectively as part of health care teams (Shannon, 1985). There is also evidence that the clinical reasoning of community-based occupational therapists is unique, and deserves emphasis in an educational curriculum (Munroe, 1996).

Practicing in the changing health care system demands acknowledgment by educational programs (Bezold, 1989; Pew Health Professions Commission, 1993). Education of occupational therapists needs to accentuate the importance of an individual's culture (Morse, 1987). The current view of disability as a function of the environment requires that therapists be prepared to analyze and facilitate function within the environment (Bowen, 1996). Health profession educators must address relevant competencies to keep up to date with the needs of American health care and the changing health care system (Bezold, 1989; Pew Health Professions Commission, 1993). The changing health care system, and the ramifications of these changes on the profession demands that educational programs focus on research training (Shannon, 1985). Education is also a possible strategy for communicating to the government, communities, and individuals the many contributions occupational therapists can make in this setting (Townsend, 1988).

METHOD

Subjects

Two hundred (200) therapists who met the inclusion criteria were randomly selected to receive the Community Practice Project (CPP) survey through the mail. The American Occupational Therapy Association registries provided lists of registered therapists practicing in Michigan, Illinois, and Indiana. Community-based practice was defined as practice where the site of intervention is in the community. Appropriate sites were identified per Moyers (1999). Home and community settings for practice included the following: home care, halfway houses, group homes, assisted living, sheltered workshops, industry and business, schools, early intervention centers, day care centers, community mental health centers, hospice, and wellness and fitness centers.

Instrument

This study was built upon the CPP (Lysack et al., 1995). The CPP survey instrument was originally developed by fourth year occupational therapy and physical therapy students at Queen's University in Kingston, Canada. Lysack et al. made revisions to the CPP survey. The final result was critiqued by an instrument expert. This survey was developed for use in Canada for comparison with Canadian educational criteria and curricula. Health care in Canada follows a socialist medicine model whereas in the United States health care is considered an industry with profit margins and cost saving measures. To be used in this study, the CPP survey needed to be revised. Changes were made to reflect the population to be studied, the United States health care system, and the use of the English language in the United States. These changes were subject to review by an author of the original study, and a face validity study. The author of the original study felt that the changes made would not alter the intent of the study. Recommendations arising from the face validity study were incorporated into the survey to increase clarity.

Data Analysis

The data gathered was analyzed dependent upon the question type. Responses to forced choice questions were entered into a computer spreadsheet program. These results were analyzed with frequency tables. These percentages were used to indicate general trends, areas of professional expertise, and other similar quantitative aspects of the study. Statistical tests were completed to determine if there were significant differences between groups. Qualitative data were analyzed for trends and used to support quantitative data.

RESULTS

Of the 200 surveys mailed to community-based therapists, 84 (42%) were returned. While this response rate is not considered excellent, it is considered adequate (Babbie, 1999). Not all respondents provided answers to every question; therefore, the total number of responses varies from question to question. Of the respondents, 65 (77%) responded to all forced choice questions. Qualitative information was provided by 72 (85%) respondents.

Profile of Respondents

The data gathered supplied a profile of the typical respondent. Table 1 provides an overview of the respondents to this survey, and those that responded to the Lysack et al. (1995) study with respect to gender, age and education. Degrees in subjects other than occupational therapy were reported by 28 (34%) of respondents. Of the respondents, 83

TABLE 1. A Percentage Comparison of Respondent Profiles (N = 83)

Category	Lysack et al.	Present Study
	Gender	
Female	99	97.5
Male	1	2.5
	Age	
20-29	21	13.3
30-39	44	14.5
40-49	23	49.4
50+	12	22.9
	Education	
Certificate in OT	–	2.4
Diploma in OT	22	0
Bachelors Degree	66	47.6
Masters Degree	10	47.6
Doctorate	2	2.4

(98.8%) were currently employed. Of the respondents, 56 (67%) reported working in one community-based position. Of the respondents, 36 (43%) have held their primary job for less than five years.

Table 2 compares the Lysack et al. respondents to the respondents of this study regarding their primary job setting, caseload, job roles and their employers' occupation. Self-employment was reported by 18 (21.3%) of respondents. A significant amount of respondents receive referrals from family physicians, 44 (53.7%), and other physicians, 36 (43.9%). There were several other referral sources of interest: (a) other health professionals, 50 (61%); (b) physical therapists, 42 (51.2%);

TABLE 2. Percentage Response of Aspects of Community Practice (N = 83)

Category	Lysack et al.	Present Study
Location		
Public School/School Board	16	59
Community/Home	48	21.7
Psychiatric Hospital	9	1.2
Caseload		
Pediatric	20	68
Adolescent	2	1.3
Adult	31	14.6
Geriatric	12	6.6
Mixed	33	9.3
Roles		
Clinician	75	90.4
Consultant, Educator	85	74.7
Administrator, Manager	30	13
Employer		
School Board/Teacher	–	39.6
Health Care Administrator	45	15.7
Government Administrator	–	12.9
Occupational Therapist	17	10

(c) occupational therapists, 29 (35.4%); and (d) school staff including administrators and teachers, 31 (38%).

Job Skills Necessary for Community-Based Practice

There were several job skills identified as necessary for practice in the community. Job skills were defined as those behavioral activities that new graduates are expected to be able to perform (Lysack et al., 1995). Respondents indicated whether their education had prepared them for specific job skills. Table 3 considers the percentages of respondents who were prepared to use a skill, who used a skill, and those who used a skill and did not feel prepared for its implementation. Table 4 lists areas of continued education and specialized techniques recommended for community-based practice.

Areas of Professional Expertise

Respondents identified several areas of professional expertise utilized in community-based practice. Professional expertise was defined as high level professional functioning acquired after knowledge and attitudes have developed with occupational therapy experience in the field (Lysack et al., 1995). It was also indicated whether they felt prepared to implement this expertise. Table 5 presents the percentage of respondents who felt prepared in an area of expertise, those who used an area, and those who used the area and did not feel prepared.

TABLE 3. Percentage Use and Preparation for Job Skills (N = 83)

Job Skill	Prepared for Use	Skill Used	Used, Not Prepared
Patient Assessment	66.3	100	33.7
Written Communication	55.4	100	45.6
Verbal Communication	49.4	97.6	49.4
Charting	62.7	86.7	33.3
Consulting	16.9	86.7	83.5
Staff Education/In-Services	31.3	85.5	–
Networking	20.5	72.3	76.7

TABLE 4. Recommended Continued Education for Community-Based Practice

Educational Area	Percent Recommended
Continued Education (N = 59)	
Sensory Integration	39
Oral-Motor Issues	20
Neurodevelopmental Treatment	19
Specialized Techniques (N = 46)	
Sensory Integration	74
Neurodevelopmental Techniques	35

TABLE 5. Percentage of Use and Preparation for Areas of Expertise (N = 80)

Area of Expertise	Prepared for Use	Skill Used	Used, Not Prepared
Self Directed Learning	40	92.5	60.8
Clinical Reasoning	66.3	86.3	34.8
Client-Centered Approach to Practice	45	85	48.5
Community Resources	26.3	71.3	71.9

DISCUSSION

Principal Roles of Community-Based Occupational Therapists

This study uncovered several significant aspects of job roles. The most common job roles were identified. Concerns about the clarity of job roles also surfaced. The implications of these concerns on the profession must be considered.

The results of this survey indicated that community-based occupational therapists frequently fill the role of clinician, and consultant/educator. The role of consultant has been extensively discussed in literature (Hurff et al., 1990; Pollack & Stewart, 1998). The role of educator is emerging in literature as important for community-based practice

(Chui, 1998; Madill et al., 1989; Teague et al., 1990). Therapists in the community are working closely with people outside the occupational therapy profession. Only 8 (10%) of respondents reported that they were employed by occupational therapists. Therapists are required to educate not only their clients, but also the health care team they are working with about occupational therapy. This necessity makes it more important that therapists have a clear understanding of what occupational therapy is and its role in treatment.

The changing health care system is demanding that allied health professionals clearly define what they will offer to clients (Bezold, 1989; Pew Health Professions Commission, 1993). Many respondents voiced concern that the role of occupational therapists in the community is determined by the therapists' interests, strengths, and understanding of occupational therapy. It was emphasized that a therapist considering this practice area needs a "clear idea how their OT skills are being used so that they are not doing someone else's job in the name of OT." This was felt to be important because "there is a lot of blurring of roles that can be difficult for young, inexperienced therapists." The potential for the blurring of job roles is considered quite high. This lack of clarity could be a significant weakness in the occupational therapy profession. If occupational therapists are unsure of their roles, they cannot clearly define their contribution to health care. Occupational therapy needs to define its role as unique and necessary (Baum & Law, 1997, 1998; Devereaux, 1991; Pew Health Professions Commission, 1993). Impressing upon occupational therapy students the role of occupational therapy in specific treatment settings could be a valuable first step toward meeting this need.

Skills and Expertise of Community-Based Occupational Therapists

The skills and expertise identified by respondents can be grouped into three categories: (a) interpersonal skills, (b) clinical skills, and (c) community specific skills.

Interpersonal skills were identified by respondents as critical for practice in this setting. A majority of respondents identified four skills and areas as necessary for community-based practice: (a) written and verbal communication, (b) consulting, (c) staff education/in-services, and (d) advocacy. This category corresponds well with the identified job roles. Working as a consultant requires that therapists be able to communicate their expertise to communities for implementation. Working as an educator similarly emphasizes the importance of coherent communication. For skills so commonly used, it is unfortunate that only around half of therapists using this skill felt prepared.

Respondents also indicated a strong need for clinical skills. More than half of respondents identified seven skills and areas of expertise as necessary for practice: (a) patient assessment, (b) charting, (c) self directed learning, (d) clinical reasoning, (e) client-centered approach to practice, (f) professional issues, and (g) use of treatment modalities. This is particularly important considering that community-based therapists frequently work independently. While the educational system is addressing these needs, there is always room for improvement. One therapist related her experience with a self-directed learning curriculum:

> I was well prepared in my education. But what was really taught was the "seek and ye shall find" curriculum. So instead of "holding our hands" and listening to students whine and complain, the "seek and ye shall find" was done. We were expected to find out [information] not just have it spooned into our brains. Now true we (all of us) were angry cause the instructors would [not] hold our hands, but we were better prepared for the complexities of OT, then and now, because we knew how to move along without handholding. We were . . . lucky to be educated back then, look at where the '60s people took OT as a profession.

A client-centered approach to treatment implies that the person and his/her environment and community are being addressed (Grady, 1995; Stancliff, 1996). Centering treatment on the client defines success as the client achieving goals he/she is interested in (Stancliff, 1996). Centering treatment on the client also implies that any lack of compliance can be interpreted as failure of the therapist to address the individual's desires and interests (Bowen, 1996; Dressler & MacRae, 1998). Abberley (1995) noted that therapists urging the individual to be the primary decision-maker incorrectly attribute failure in treatment to the individual's lack of motivation, the lack of support within the health care system, and various other areas. This error suggested a professional failure where occupational therapists were not successfully implementing the principles of client-centered treatment (Abberley, 1995).

A final area of expertise included community specific skills. A majority of respondents indicated that six skills and expertise were important for community-based practice: (a) networking, (b) community resources, (c) management of volunteers, (d) program evaluation,

(e) health promotion/disease prevention, and (f) multicultural practice issues. Knowledge in these areas can serve to tailor a program to the needs of a community. Understanding the community resources available, and having the networking abilities to recruit assistance should facilitate agreement between a community's needs and resources and the implementation of community-based programs. Health promotion and disease prevention programs require the participation of the community to succeed. Program development and evaluation should be structured to keep the community involved. The idea of health promotion has been present in occupational therapy literature as early as the 1960s. Health promotion has been a topic for many leaders in the occupational therapy profession who promote the concept as beneficial to society and a good fit for occupational therapy (Finlayson & Edwards, 1995; West, 1967; White, 1986). Allied health professions, such as occupational therapy, practicing health promotion and disease prevention in the community offer cost effective solutions to the dilemmas of health care management (Beech et al., 1999; Chui, 1998). Multiculturalism is important in a community-based setting as the influence of culture is increasingly recognized (Grady, 1995; Morse, 1987; Townsend, 1987). Therapists must incorporate culture if they are to successfully create intervention programs that are meaningful for the community (Morse, 1987).

Group Effects on Skills and Areas of Expertise Identification

The profile of respondents showed two potential groupings: (1) bachelors' and master's degrees as highest level of education; and (2) school occupational therapists, and those working outside of the school. Statistical tests were used to explore these groupings. The number of respondents whose highest educational level was a bachelor's degree was equal to the number of respondents whose highest educational level was a master's degree. There were no significant differences between these two groups ($p = .05$) when considering job skills, and areas of expertise identified as prepared for, or necessary. A little more than half of respondents primarily worked in a school or for a school board. The responses of school based therapists were significantly different, in three areas, from the responses of therapists working in other locations. School therapists reported using different skills ($p = .004$). Therapists in the school differed on the skills they felt prepared to use ($p = .05$). These therapists differed on the areas of expertise they used in practice ($p = .10$). It is possible that these differences altered the results of the study.

Education Issues

Townsend (1988) stated that education about community-based practice is the core factor in preparing occupational therapists for community contributions. Pimentel and Ryan (1996) found that none of their subjects felt that community-based practice had been covered adequately in college. Lysack et al. (1995) identified a need for better preparation for community-based practice. Lysack et al. indicated that 85% of community-based therapists felt that continued education was necessary to meet the needs of their position. Of respondents to this current study, 75 (91%) felt that continued education was necessary for practice in this area.

There were several skills and areas of professional expertise identified as necessary for practice that therapists were not prepared for through their formal education. Respondents to this current survey were concerned about a lack of preparation for the following skills: (a) consulting, (b) networking, (c) staff education/in-services, (d) verbal communication and (e) written communication. Respondents to this survey identified these areas of professional expertise as not adequately covered in their formal education: (a) community resources, (b) self-directed learning, (c) client-centered approach to practice and (d) advocacy.

Education of occupational therapists must address skills and expertise needed for community-based practice. The traditional education of heath care professionals is appropriate for the roles and responsibilities that will be encountered in traditional health care (Bowen, 1996; Peat, 1991). McColl (1998) stated that occupational therapists need to be prepared to work within the confines and expectations of community-based practice. Peat (1991) stated that "[h]ealth professionals must receive special training on professional roles appropriate for community programmes [sic]" (p. 232). Identifying which skills and areas of expertise beginning therapists are not adequately prepared for could be the first step to providing complete educational programs.

Fieldwork Suggestions

Several issues were raised concerning fieldwork. With the increased interest in community-based practice, many respondents were being contacted to provide fieldwork experiences. These opportunities are frequently economically and logistically unfeasible. However, therapists in this area did not encourage the development of fieldwork in community-based settings. One respondent stated that "a student must have core treatment experiences in traditional settings, e.g., acute or rehab hospitals before venturing out into often unstructured treatment settings." Another respondent felt that "students would really benefit from more exposure to real-world OT practices. Perhaps with brief observations, or even on videotape," instead of fieldwork placements. Therapists also suggested that the area is so specialized that training can only be received on the job.

Research Concerns

The need for community-based therapists to adopt the role of researcher has been greatly emphasized in the literature (McColl, 1998; Nelson, 1997; West, 1967). However, this current research indicated that only 2 (2.3%) respondents fill the role of researcher. Further, 11 (13.3%) respondents reported they used the skills of a researcher while 42 (50.6%) reported that these skills were not relevant. Respondents were cognizant of the need for more awareness of the occupational therapy profession to "increase physician referral for appropriate clients." Several respondents noted that occupational therapy needed to be promoted as a viable profession in this setting, but did not suggest methods for accomplishing this.

Limitations

This study has several limitations which include (a) the lack of a second mailing, (b) a purposive sampling area, (c) the focus of the survey and (d) the survey instrument used.

This research project did not include a mechanism for a second mailing. Had this been included, it is possible a higher response rate could have been achieved. A higher response rate would give the data collected more credibility as representing the thoughts of community-based therapists.

The therapists selected for this survey were from specific states. Due to this narrow geographic area, the responses cannot be generalized to all community-based therapists practicing in the United States.

The focus of the CPP survey was on the link between job skills, professional expertise, and educational preparation (Lysack et al., 1995). This focus has inherent assumptions that must be considered. The ability of professional occupational therapy curricula to address the needs of respondents must be considered.

A final limitation concerns the formation and structure of the survey. The CPP survey was developed in late 1991 and 1992 with a perspective that was current for that time (Lysack et al., 1995). As Lysack et al. state, the area of practice has become much more dynamic since then. Another limitation is that the CPP survey lacked clarity. Several respondents avoided answering questions noting that they did not understand the questions. A final limitation with the survey is that several questions were not included. The survey did not separate therapists with an entry level master's degree from therapists with an advanced master's degree. The survey failed to identify the occupational therapy programs respondents had attended. The survey also failed to identify the year that therapists graduated from their occupational therapy program. Another valuable question not included in the survey was the number of years the respondents have practiced.

CONCLUSIONS

The aim of this research was to identify job roles, job skills, and professional expertise in community-based practice. It was also interested in assessing the educational preparation of therapists for practice in this area. The findings of this study have satisfied these expectations.

This study provided much information. The study developed a profile of the typical respondent, their job roles, skills, and areas of professional expertise. There were two significant findings of this study regarding job roles. The first is the large potential for blurring professional roles. The second is the tendency for job roles to conform to the interests and expertise of a particular therapist. Significant findings of this study regarding job skills were that networking, consulting, and communication skills were areas that are not adequately addressed in curricula. Significant findings of this study regarding professional expertise were that community resources, self directed learning, and client-centered approach to practice were areas that need more attention in curricula.

In general, respondents were positive about working in community-based settings. As one respondent noted, "I have loved working in the school community . . . OT is absolutely a wonderful career."

REFERENCES

Abberley, P. (1995). Disabling ideology in health and welfare–the case of occupational therapy. *Disability & Society, 10,* 221-232.
Adamson, B., Sinclair-Legge, G., Cusick, A., & Nordholm, L. (1994). Attitudes, values and orientation to professional practice: A study of Australian occupational therapists. *British Journal of Occupational Therapy, 57,* 476-480.

Babbie, E. (1990). *Survey research methods* (2nd ed.). Belmont, CA: Wadsworth Publishing Company.

Baum, C., & Law, M. (1997). Occupational therapy practice: Focusing on occupational performance. *American Journal of Occupational Therapy, 51,* 277-288.

Baum, C., & Law, M. (1998). Community health: A responsibility, an opportunity, and a fit for occupational therapy. *American Journal of Occupational Therapy, 52,* 7-10.

Beech, R., Rudd, A., Tilling, K., & Wolfe, C. (1999). Economic consequences of early inpatient discharge to community-based rehabilitation for stroke in an inner-London teaching hospital. *Stroke, 30,* 729-735.

Bezold, L. (1989). The future of health care: Implications for the allied health professions. *Journal of Allied Health, 18,* 437-457.

Bowen, R. (1996, May). Practicing what we preach: Embracing the independent living movement. *OT Practice, 1(5),* 20-24.

Chui, D. (1998). What is community-based rehabilitation: An implication of the roles of community occupational therapists in Hong Kong. *Occupational Therapy in Health Care, 11,* 79-98.

Devereaux, E. (1991). The issue is–Community-based practice. *American Journal of Occupational Therapy, 45,* 944-946.

Dressler, J., & MacRae, A. (1998). Advocacy, partnerships, and client-centered practice in California. *Occupational Therapy in Mental Health, 14,* 35-43.

Finlayson, M., & Edwards, J. (1995). Integrating the concepts of health promotion and community into occupational therapy practice. *Canadian Journal of Occupational Therapy, 62,* 70-75.

Grady, A. (1995). Building inclusive community: A challenge for occupational therapy. *American Journal of Occupational Therapy, 49,* 300-310.

Hurff, J., Lowe, H., Ho, B., & Hoffman, N. (1990). Networking: A successful linkage for community occupational therapists. *American Journal of Occupational Therapy, 44,* 424-430.

Lysack, C., Stadnyk, R., Paterson, M., McLeod, K., & Krefting, L. (1995). Professional expertise of occupational therapists in community practice: Results of an Ontario survey. *Canadian Journal of Occupational Therapy, 62,* 138-147.

Madill, H., Townsend, E., & Schultz, P. (1989). Implementing a health promotion strategy in occupational therapy education and practice. *American Journal of Occupational Therapy, 56,* 67-72.

McColl, M. (1998). What do we need to know to practice occupational therapy in the community? *American Journal of Occupational Therapy, 52,* 11-18.

Morse, A. (1987). A cultural intervention model for developmentally disabled adults: An expanded role for occupational therapy. *Occupational Therapy in Health Care, 4,* 103-114.

Moyers, P. (1999). The Guide to Occupational Therapy Practice [Special issue]. *American Journal of Occupational Therapy, 53*(3).

Munroe, H. (1996). Clinical reasoning in community occupational therapy. *British Journal of Occupational Therapy, 59,* 196-202.

Nelson, D. (1997). Why the profession of occupational therapy will flourish in the 21st century. *American Journal of Occupational Therapy, 51,* 11-24.

Peat, M. (1991). Community-based rehabilitation–development and structure: Part 2. *Clinical Rehabilitation, 5,* 231-239.

Pew Health Professions Commission. (1993). *Health professions education for the future: Schools in service to the nation.* San Fransisco, CA: Pew Health Professions Commission.

Pimentel, S., & Ryan, S. (1996). Working with clients with learning disabilities and multiple physical handicaps: A comparison between hospital and community-based therapists. *British Journal of Occupational Therapy, 59,* 313-318.

Pollack, N., & Stewart, D. (1998). Occupational performance needs of school aged children with physical disabilities in the community. *Physical & Occupational Therapy in Pediatrics, 18,* 55-68.

Renwick, R., Cockburn, L., Colantonio, A., & Friedland, J. (1996). Preparing students for practice in a changing community environment: An innovative course. *Occupational Therapy International, 3,* 262-273.

Shannon, P. (1985). From another perspective: An overview of the issue. *Occupational Therapy in Health Care, 2,* 3-11.

Stancliff, B. (1996, July). Helping others achieve their goals. *OT Practice, 1(7),* 13-16.

Strickland, L. (1991). Directions for the future–Occupational therapy practice then and now. 1949-the present. *American Journal of Occupational Therapy, 45,* 105-107.

Teague, M., Cipriano, R., & McGhee, V. (1990). Health promotion as a rehabilitation service for people with disabilities. *Journal of Rehabilitation, 56,* 52-56.

Townsend, E. (1987). Strategies for community occupational therapy program development. *Canadian Journal of Occupational Therapy, 54,* 65-70.

Townsend, E. (1988). Developing community occupational therapy services in Canada. *Canadian Journal of Occupational Therapy, 52,* 69-74.

Vanier, C., & Hebert, M. (1995). An occupational therapy course on community practice. *Canadian Journal of Occupational Therapy, 62,* 76-81.

West, W. (1967). The occupational therapists changing responsibility to the community. *American Journal of Occupational Therapy, 2,* 312-316.

White, V. (1986). Promoting health and wellness: A theme for the eighties. *American Journal of Occupational Therapy, 40,* 743-748.

The Pizzi Holistic Wellness Assessment

Michael Pizzi, MS, OTR/L, CHES, FAOTA

SUMMARY. This paper describes the Pizzi Holistic Wellness Assessment tool. Using theory from the field of health promotion and expertise gained in his private home health practice, the author developed and pilot tested this assessment on a variety of individuals. The assessment is designed to be used with different populations in a variety of settings to help clients self assess their health and well-being. *[Article copies available for a fee from The Haworth Document Delivery Service: 1-800-342-9678. E-mail address: <getinfo@haworthpressinc.com> Website: <http://www.HaworthPress.com> © 2001 by The Haworth Press, Inc. All rights reserved.]*

KEYWORDS. Wellness, wellness assessment, health promotion

We must recognize the responsibility of the profession to change with changing demands for its services, to adapt via new approaches, to assume different roles, to develop the preparation for them, and to recruit in a new mold rather than by recasting the prototype of an earlier time. (West, 1967, p. 175)

Michael Pizzi is Clinical Assistant Professor, Sacred Heart University/Department of Occupational Therapy, Fairfield, CT 06850 (E-mail: mpizzi5857@aol.com).

The author thanks the many people who have used the tool clinically for their feedback. Additional thanks to the students and faculty of Ithaca College OT Department for helpful input, Peggy Wittman, EdD, OTR, FAOTA, for constructive assistance and her friendship and Amy Darragh, MS, OTR for her supportive feedback.

The Pizzi Holistic Wellness Assessment is protected by copyright and is reproduced here with permission of the author. No reproduction of any kind or use of the tool is permitted without express written consent of the author.

[Haworth co-indexing entry note]: "The Pizzi Holistic Wellness Assessment." Pizzi, Michael. Co-published simultaneously in *Occupational Therapy in Health Care* (The Haworth Press, Inc.) Vol. 13, No. 3/4, 2001, pp. 51-66; and: *Community Occupational Therapy Education and Practice* (eds: Beth P. Velde, and Peggy Prince Wittman) The Haworth Press, Inc., 2001, pp. 51-66. Single or multiple copies of this article are available for a fee from The Haworth Document Delivery Service [1-800-342-9678, 9:00 a.m. - 5:00 p.m. (EST). E-mail address: getinfo@haworthpressinc.com].

Concepts of wellness and health promotion and disease prevention were embraced by early founders, philosophers, and theorists in occupational therapy. Meyer (1922) called for a balance of work, rest, sleep and play so that people can live well and be productive. He viewed mental illness as a disorder in living and was a proponent of occupation as the central concept in helping to facilitate order. He also wrote that "man learns to organize time and he does so in terms of doing things" (p. 6), alluding to the fact that when an individual is not actively engaged in meaningful productive occupation, he/she becomes, or has potential to become, disorganized in life and lose a sense of time, routine and habit.

Slagle (1922) developed the concept that habits and routines of daily living help people to organize daily life and daily occupations and proposed that a breakdown of habits and routines can lead to disorder and illness in one's life. She discussed how occupational therapists would utilize 'habit training' to return a person to healthier living:

> . . . for the most part, our lives are made up of habit reactions. Occupation used remedially serves to overcome some habits, to modify others and construct new ones, to the end that habit reaction will be favorable to the restoration and maintenance of health. (Slagle, 1922, p. 14)

Occupation was seen as the ends as well as the means to rehabilitate and habilitate individuals and to empower them towards healthy living and the development of healthy lifestyles.

In addition to its focus on activity, the profession of occupational therapy has always been known for its emphasis on integration and awareness of body, mind and, more recently, spiritual aspects of health; and how the interrelatedness of these factors impacts a person's ability to carry out daily routines and occupations. Occupational therapy was encouraged over three decades ago to create opportunities where well-being can be realized for all people and to develop new roles for therapists in the area of wellness and health promotion. Speaking of these issues at an AOTA conference, West (1967) stated:

> [There is a] repeated emphasis on health, as well as illness, on prevention of disease and disability, in addition to seeking the cures not yet discovered, on promotion of well-being, not just being satisfied that there is an absence of infirmity, on continuity of care . . . and on comprehensive health services . . . the trends in these direc-

tions are unmistakable. They are also irreversible. To recognize them, however, is only the first step. We must also interpret their meaning for each of our specialty areas and aggressively adapt or redesign our roles to provide a more viable future service. (p. 178)

Kielhofner and Burke (1983) also noted that the profession of occupational therapy was based on "a broad appreciation of the occupational nature of human beings, their mind-body unity, their self-maintenance through occupation, and the dynamic rhythm and balance of their organized behavior . . ." (p. 31). Current trends in occupational therapy emphasize a return to occupation and to the integration of well-being and occupation into daily practice (Moyers, 1999, 2000).

Related to these beliefs, occupational therapy is becoming a leading force in client-centered care and the major proponent of the importance of meaning in the being and doing of daily living. Clinicians can begin to facilitate this for each client and can promote well-being by (1) providing occupational choices, (2) respecting autonomy and control over the doing process, (3) collaborating rather than dictating what wellness should look like to individuals and, most importantly, (4) addressing the issue of body, mind and spirit unity and (5) having an appreciation for a systems perspective of health.

GUIDING PRINCIPLES OF WELLNESS

Wellness has been defined by many health professionals to generally mean a state of optimized health satisfying to the individual. Dunn (1954), a physician, was one of the first to conceptualize and define wellness as an integrated method of behaving which is oriented toward maximizing the potential the individual is capable of within the environment where he/she is functioning. From this conceptualization, it can be assumed that Dunn envisioned wellness as a program of care (method) and not simply a concept. He also takes a very holistic occupation-centered approach in his definition and clearly sees the interplay between person and environment.

Opatz (1985) views wellness as the process of adapting patterns of behavior so that they lead to improved health and heightened life satisfaction. Hettler (1990) defines wellness as an "active process through which individuals become aware of and make choices toward a more successful existence" (p. 1111).

According to Dossey and Guzetta (1989),

> This health model [of wellness] assumes that every individual has innate capacities for healing, nurturing, self reflection, taking risks, and for making change toward wellness; that all people are searching for answers about the life process, meaning, and purpose; and that health is also about individuals being able to live according to their own beliefs. (pp. 69-70)

There have been numerous references in the occupational therapy literature regarding the concept of wellness. These include an examination of the balance of work, rest, sleep and play (Meyer, 1922); examining perceptions about time and degrees of harmony or conflict in our unique configuration of goal directed activities (Christiansen, 2000); balance, value, meaning and being client centered which contributes to health and well-being (Johnson, 1993); and the idea that engagement in occupation contributes to and influences health (Reilly, 1962). More recently, wellness and health promotion have been included in the Occupational Therapy Guide to Practice (Moyers, 1999) as a major area for intervention. However, before an occupational therapist can intervene, he/she must be able to evaluate based on some guiding principles.

Christiansen and Baum (1991) summarize general beliefs and values that influence occupational therapy and incorporate the philosophy of wellness. These beliefs include:

1. Engagement in occupation is of value because it provides opportunities for individuals to influence their well-being by gaining fulfillment in living.
2. Through the experience of occupation or doing, the individual is able to achieve mastery and competence by learning skills and strategies necessary for coping with problems and adapting to limitations.
3. As competence is gained and autonomy can be expressed, independence can be achieved.
4. Autonomy implies choice and control over environmental circumstances, thus opportunities for exerting self determination should be reflected in intervention strategies.
5. An individual's choice and control extend to decisions about intervention, thus occupational therapy is identified as a collaborative

process between the therapist and recipient of care whose values are respected.

6. Because of occupational therapy's focus on life performance, it is neither somatic nor psychological, but concerned with the unity of body and mind in doing. (p. 9)

Pizzi (1997) developed a set of guiding principles in wellness and health promotion which he incorporated into continuing education workshops and in his clinical practice. These principles (Pizzi, 1996) are used to holistically assess and treat all individuals and their caregivers (primarily adults but applicable, with adaptation, to infants, children and adolescents). Pizzi uses the term 'activity' purposefully since the continuing education workshops are interdisciplinary and the term 'occupation' would apply primarily only to occupational therapy. These principles are:

1. Engaging in life activity is health promoting.
2. Activity must be of a person's interest and have meaning to the individual to effectively promote wellness.
3. A loving and supportive environment promotes health and wellness.
4. Adaptation in life to accommodate new changes that occur in health contributes to well-being and life satisfaction.
5. Being productive, vital and a contribution to others is health promoting.
6. People must make an active choice to live well and be responsible for their choices.
7. Open and honest communications are health promoting and contribute to wellness.
8. Life affirming and self affirming actions and words promote positive healthful living and wellness. (Pizzi, 1997, p. 17)

These guiding principles can be integrated and utilized in community centered care and applied to all ages and diagnostic groups including traditional rehabilitation programs.

THE PIZZI HOLISTIC WELLNESS ASSESSMENT (PHWA)

Before holistic wellness interventions can be effective, therapists must assess a person's level of well-being while engaged in client-centered and occupation-based practice. When therapists are both client and occupation centered, facilitation of wellness becomes a natural extension and a vital part of the occupational therapy process. This can and must occur in all environments where an occupational therapist or occupational therapy assistant practices the art and science of occupational therapy. Wellness includes both remediating and preventing a breakdown of daily habits, routines, occupations, and meaning in people's lives.

This potential or real "breakdown" of daily living activity performance can include every activity meaningful to a person with any deficit in any area. An individual with arthritis that causes immobility and therefore impaired ability to shop, and a busy homemaker/worker with no medical, physical or psychosocial diagnosis trying to balance several roles, are both examples of people experiencing breakdowns in activity patterns. Frank (2000) states:

> Persons must cope with feelings of frustration when their ability to perform daily activities breaks down. They experience anger and frustration over loss of control. They suffer feelings about being helpless and dependent on others. They feel distress and guilt about added family responsibilities. (p. 27)

According to the ICIDH-2 Classification System (Moyers, 1999), these breakdowns in daily living may be categorized under impairments, activity limitations or participation restrictions. Concurrently with the use of this revised classification system, it is vital to create new paradigms of health which incorporate community, client and occupation centered assessments and interventions. Jackson (1999) advocates for development of more client centered self assessments, stating that there is a huge gap in the allied health professions, especially occupational therapy, in the area of assessment that actually considers clients' own self perceptions of their health and the meaning they assign to occupations and routines of daily living.

To date, this author uncovered no known formal and documented assessments in the allied health fields that are (a) conceptually holistic, (b) wellness based, (c) client centered, and (d) self-administered (Hemphill-Pearson, 1999; Marcus, 1999; Van Deusen & Brunt, 1997). The Canadian Occupational Performance Measure (COPM) (Law, Baptiste, McColl, Opzoomer, Palatajko, & Pollock, 1990) is the closest to being a holistic wellness client centered assessment; however, it is not self administered and is used only by occupational therapists.

The Pizzi Holistic Wellness Assessment was developed from an interdisciplinary perspective (although very much occupationally derived) that emphasizes self-perceptions of health and strategies for self-responsibility facilitated by therapists. The author has long believed that allied health professionals, including occupational therapy, often do not incorporate the goals, beliefs, values, attitudes and meaningful needs of the client being served. Over time, in his community centered practice, the author recognized that people were much more motivated in therapy when he initiated treatment with at least one occupational activity important to the client. Reductionistic (e.g., range of motion, strengthening, cognitive, perceptual) treatment was incorporated into the occupational activity and not worked on separately, creating a holistic framework from which the client could gain skills integrated into some meaningful productive daily living occupation.

The Pizzi Holistic Wellness Assessment (PHWA) is a self assessment designed to assist individuals to become aware of the most important health issues affecting daily occupational performance. The assessment also addresses self responsibility for health by exploring self determined strategies to optimize health. Therapists are only facilitators of health and wellness. They do not do things to or for people, but rather suggest ways to optimize healthy living and facilitate the process of health and healing by increasing awareness to issues (physical, psychosocial and environmental) that need to be addressed. Even when it appears that a specific treatment positively changes occupational performance, the aspects of wellness and health and healing occur when the person is led to self discovery on how to best manage that aspect of his/her being. After self-discovery, the therapy process unfolds collaboratively between client and therapist.

Another objective of the Pizzi Holistic Wellness Assessment is for therapists to obtain the self perception of the client in eight areas of health. Operational definitions of these areas emphasize occupational activity and the doing process. These eight areas were developed based on interdisciplinary literature (Ader, Felton & Cohen, 1991; Benson & Stark, 1996; Bruner, 1990; Capra, 1982; Christiansen & Baum, 1993; Csikszentmihalyi, 1990, 1993; Ferguson, 1980; Johnson, 1986, 1993; Kalat, 1998; Law, 1998; Law et al., 1990; Moyers, 1993; Neistadt & Crepeau, 1998; Pauls & Reed, 1996; Pert, 1997; Reed, 1991; Ryan & Travis, 1991; Weil, 1995; Zemke & Clark, 1996).

The Pizzi Holistic Wellness Assessment is based on the wellness principles stated above and principles of general systems theory (von Bertalanffy, 1968). The application of systems thinking (particularly an open system) to occupational therapy examines the interrelationship between the environment and the person. It also examines the various systems of the person and emphasizes that if there is a breakdown or dysfunction in one system, it will have an impact on other systems. For example, a person who experiences a cerebral vascular accident (CVA) may also experience deficits in the psychosocial area of health (e.g., depression, sadness, anger, guilt for poor health habits). While most therapists assume this often occurs, the clinical experience of the author suggests both physical and psychosocial rehabilitation (or interventions) are not formally addressed simultaneously in occupational therapy by either standardized or non-standardized assessments. Yet, a person with CVA and possible psychosocial deficits will most likely experience motivational problems and feel a loss of meaning in daily living, which can then affect traditional physical rehabilitation. Bateson (1996) supports this idea and discusses how occupation, when delivered in appropriate occupational contexts, can have multiple positive impacts when used therapeutically.

Unfortunately, many therapists may not have a means by which the psychosocial impairments and physical impairments can be addressed. In addition, without formal documentation of the psychosocial impairments, therapists are often limited in the scope of treatment that will be reimbursed, even though psychosocial interventions are within the scope of occupational therapy practice and are often reimbursable when progress is demonstrated via improved occupational performance.

Holistic clinical reasoning is often a skill developed by more experienced practitioners. Standardized assessments often provide practical objective data that is more in the procedural realm of information. However, as Mattingly and Fleming (1993) point out, "When practitioners rely exclusively on procedural reasoning, they are likely to focus their treatment on performance components rather than life tasks" (p. 47). The Pizzi Holistic Wellness Assessment, via client narrative, examines multiple areas of health as they affect occupational performance. Therapists and clients using this assessment can become more acutely aware of the multidimensional aspects of health and the interrelatedness of the physical, psychosocial, spiritual and environmental aspects of health. Furthermore, it enables therapists to set treatment priorities and develop a wellness plan with strategies that are meaningful to the client. Objective and non-medical problems and deficits are discovered after the administration of the Pizzi Holistic Wellness Assessment. The assessment also focuses on subjective self-assessment narrative to explore the root of a deficit as well as strategies for intervention that are both subjective (from the client) and objective (from the therapist/wellness expert).

ADMINISTRATION
OF THE PIZZI HOLISTIC WELLNESS ASSESSMENT

The assessment is depicted as a circle, symbolically demonstrating that all areas of health interrelate and affect each other. The client is instructed to rate each of eight areas of health from 0-10 on a rating line with tic marks noting 0 (poor health) to 10 (excellent health). The instruction is: "Rate yourself from 0 (poor health) to 10 (excellent health) in each of these 8 areas. Use your gut reaction as you rate yourself, as that is your true feeling of your level of well-being in that particular area. Later you will be able to discuss each one separately and tell me more about your rating."

Following the overall rating of health, each of the eight areas are separated for a more comprehensive client centered narrative. Within each section, four occupationally focused questions are asked of the client. These questions are:

1. What are the factors in my life that caused me to rate this area as I did?
2. What are the (specific health area) problems that I am experiencing?
3. How do these problems affect my day to day activities?
4. How can I overcome these problems?

These questions were developed to assess various areas of function and to provide therapists with data that may not be obtained in a traditional format of interview or through standardized assessment. This data includes: (a) client self-awareness of health issues, (b) insight into personal levels of health, wellness and illness, (c) client insight into other factors having an impact on one's health in a particular area, (d) awareness of the impact of a certain level of wellness on daily occupations and their performance. Question 4 has been one of the most crucial in data collection. The answer illustrates for therapists whether clients have the ability to problem solve and be adaptive enough to engage in self responsibility for personal health and well-being.

Once these individual sheets are completed, the therapist gathers the information, and, along with data from pertinent and relevant other formal or informal assessments if needed, works in collaboration with the client (and significant others if decided upon by therapist and client) to develop wellness interventions for improved health, health behavior change, or to balance one's life. Unlike a test of strength, endurance, cognitive perceptual, activities of daily living, or mood/affect, this assessment immediately directs the therapist to the arena of health and development of well-being instead of reducing health and occupational activity to their components. These reductionistic components of health are integrated with the daily living deficits affected by health problems self-determined by the client.

VALIDITY AND RELIABILITY

A panel of experts from occupational therapy, physical therapy, nursing, holistic health, health education and social work examined the assessment and concurred regarding the compatibility of the PWHA with the theoretical and philosophical framework from which it was derived. After each of these experts self administered the assessment, there was agreement on the eight specific areas of health that comprise the assessment. It was also agreed that the four occupational questions within each category gather relevant qualitative data from which wellness interventions can be planned. Currently, the tool has face and content validity. It has been used successfully as a clinical tool with populations ranging from post baccalaureate level occupational therapy students, the well elderly, individuals with mild dementia and their caregivers, people with HIV and terminal illness, and with college students with no identified occupational activity deficits. Currently, using qualitative methods, research is being conducted on development of themes of wellness utilizing this tool in several different populations. More research needs to be undertaken to develop reliability and to further validate this tool.

The qualitative data that this tool obtains includes the multidimensional self-described factors of deficits in well-being that are relevant to the field of occupational therapy, especially as the profession of occupational therapy further embraces the need for occupational histories and narratives of clients. The richness of this data provides information specific to the client's life and lifestyle different from data normally retrieved from non-wellness centered assessments and interviews. This allows therapists to view the person as an individual, creating a client centered approach with a personal health story and narrative, and further humanizes the therapy and health care experience for people.

CASE EXAMPLES

Bill is a 22-year-old physical therapy student. In the physical branch of the assessment, his self-rating was a 9. "I feel that I am pretty healthy. I play sports 5-6 times a week and lift weights or jog. My major problem is motivation to exercise more. I used to play soccer and now I do not, so I have gained some weight, which is just not me to not be fit." The therapist who assessed this rather 'well' client stated that she felt the client was self-conscious about his physique, given his mention of this problem three times in five minutes when she interviewed him after he filled out the assessment. After careful probing in this area, the therapist also discovered that the client had thoracic outlet syndrome causing pain and discomfort in his wrist and shoulder, which he attributed to playing volleyball. The pain also affected occupational functioning as a student. "My wrist has a noticeable affect on daily activity. For instance, this is only the third section of the first question on this assessment, and I have already rested my wrist twice. It does affect my note taking in class and in performing some manual therapy techniques."

This example is provided to demonstrate that, despite a self perceived high level of wellness (rating self a 9/10), the client experienced moderate impairment in occupations related to leisure and his role of student. The discussion after the client's self rating affords therapists the opportunity to collect data that the client may not have discussed. An open-ended interview supplements the client narrative.

The Pizzi Holistic Wellness Assessment is useful across all diagnostic groups, with significant others (the tool has been adapted by the author for the significant other/caregiver/family) and with adults over the age of 18 (on whom it has been currently tested). For people with cognitive impairments, modifications have been made to elicit relevant wellness data (e.g., using other key words or phrases to elicit narrative versus using solely the rating scale of 0-10). Caregivers are also asked to provide data on the client using the assessment and to provide data on themselves for therapists to examine the impact of a person's illness/wellness on the caregiving situation. This has been used successfully with caregivers of people with dementia who have discovered several alternative coping strategies, were able to develop more adaptive styles of caregiving and became more aware of the need for balance of occupations in their own lives. After administration and interpretation with one caregiver, she stated:

I knew that I needed to take better care of myself. My husband's illness has taken its toll on me and I have given up everything because I feel guilty and ashamed if I do anything I like for myself. I see now why I feel that way, and how much I can actually do if I just make a new little routine for myself that includes time for me. I also see which areas of my life [health] I am doing better in and which areas I have to do better at. I definitely need to have card parties again!

The occupational therapist then worked with her on developing a routine that included all the caregiver responsibilities as well as leisure and self maintenance occupations, and helped her develop an awareness, through education, about the impact of each health area on overall health. She self-identified where she needed support and developed a plan on how to ask for support. Over time, the occupational therapist perceived a more alive and vivacious woman who exclaimed (when this was pointed out), " I actually feel like a new person since I see that being well is not just a physical thing."

In pediatrics, this tool is an excellent addition to assess caregiver burden and stress when dealing with a family system containing a disabled client. For example, one mother of a child with autism responded to her assessment results by paying more attention to her other children when she recognized that her area of family was including, at least emotionally, only she and her child with autism. She was spending so much time with the child she began to neglect her 'family system.' It can also be used for older children without cognitive impairment to help them better develop wellness lifestyles while coping with a physical or psychosocial impairment.

A father who came to the author for a wellness consultation realized that his personal issues around food, which led to increasing problems with weight, breathing, and circulation, influenced his 10-year-old who was developing similar food habits. Intervention on a number of levels (family, psychosocial, spiritual, physical and occupational) led to improved nutrition and a more balanced lifestyle. He felt he became a more positive role model for his son, and he began to spend less time in his 'workaholic lifestyle' and more time with his family. After six months, he and his son became more physically fit and active, a health goal this man set for himself. This also resonated in his improved posture and a more positive affect.

Persons using the PHWA as a clinical tool found it to be very revealing about self-perceptions of health. It also validated for many that they cope well in daily occupational situations when previously they felt they had not coped well. Others stated that they had much more awareness of how one area of health definitely had an impact on others. This led them to alter life patterns and habits that subsequently led to improved health and well-being in all areas. Future research regarding this assessment will address specific populations, examine themes of wellness, and explore how this tool can easily be integrated into all practice arenas.

CONCLUSION

There is a great need for subjective, client centered assessments in the allied health professions, particularly in occupational therapy. Assessments which target only objective and physical data reduce the client to a set of physical deficits to be remediated, and dehumanize the person being served. In allied health, and particularly in occupational therapy, there are no formal and documented wellness, prevention or health promotion assessments, and none proclaiming they are client centered and self-administered. Occupational performance must begin to include examination of health and wellness, and to explore more ways those areas can be assessed and evaluated while maintaining a client centered and occupation focus.

The Pizzi Holistic Wellness Assessment can be used with all populations, and can be incorporated into entrepreneurial practices, community centered care, traditional therapy programs and with workplace specific practice. It is the first allied health self-assessment that aims at the total integration of mind, body and spirit and the physical, psychosocial and environmental domains of health. It also focuses therapists on immediate concerns of clients and caregivers, on what is most meaningful in a client's life, and what resources the client or caregiver possesses to approach and follow up with health interventions. Importantly, given the current health care system and a focus on managed care, the assessment assists clients in exploring their own strengths and resources that self-determine how behavioral change, in the area of occupational performance, can be made and implemented. Therapists of the future will be consultants and facilitators of health. They will be entrepreneurs exploring innovative strategies to access the health care system and develop caring and humanitarian wellness based programs. The Pizzi Holistic Wellness Assessment contributes to and enhances those roles for therapists. It is a tool for educators to incorporate into curricula for courses on community centered practice. Further reliability and validity studies are needed; however, it has been demonstrated that the Pizzi Holistic Wellness Assessment is very effective in developing clinical wellness interventions.

> How can you get very far?
> If you don't know Who you Are?
> How can you do what you ought,
> If you don't know What you Got?
> And if you don't know Which to Do
> Of all the things in front of you
> Then what you'll have in front of you
> Is just a mess without a clue
> Of all the best that can come true
> If you know What and Which and Who

> *–The Tao of Pooh* (Hoff, 1982, p. 58)

NOTE

Further clarification about the assessment and inquiries into its integration into curriculums, practice settings and its use in developing wellness programs and workshops can be addressed to Michael Pizzi, 10 Wall Street #209, Norwalk, CT 06852, or e-mail at <mpizzi5857@aol.com> or <pizzim@sacredheart.edu>.

REFERENCES

Ader, R., Felton, D. & Cohen, N. (1991). *Psychoneuroimmunology* (2nd Ed.). San Diego: Academic Press.

Bateson, M.C. (1996). Enfolded activity and the concept of occupation. In R. Zemke and F. Clark (Eds). *Occupational science: The evolving discipline.* Philadelphia: F.A. Davis.

Benson, H. & Stark, M. (1996). *Timeless healing: The power and biology of belief.* New York: Scribner.

Bruner, J. (1990). *Acts of meaning.* Cambridge, MA: Harvard University Press.

Capra, F.T. (1982). *The turning point: Science, society and the rising culture.* New York: Bantam.

Christiansen, C. & Baum, C. (Eds.) (1991). *Occupational therapy: Overcoming human performance deficits.* Thorofare, NJ: Slack.

Christiansen, C. (Ed.) (2000). *Ways of living.* Bethesda, MD: American Occupational Therapy Association.

Csikszentmihalyi, M. (1990). *Flow*. New York: Harper Collins Publishers.
Csikszentmihalyi, M. (1993). *The evolving self: A psychology for the third millennium*. New York: Harper Collins Publishers.
Dossey, B.M. & Guzzetta, C. E. (1989). Wellness, values clarification and motivation. In B.M. Dossey (Ed.). *Holistic health promotion: A guide for practice*. Rockville, MD: Aspen Publishers.
Dunn, H. (1954). *High level wellness*. Arlington, VA: R.W. Beatty.
Ferguson, M. (1980*). The aquarian conspiracy: Personal and social transformation in the 1980's*. Los Angeles, CA: Tarcher, Inc.
Frank, G. (2000). *The meaning of selfcare occupations*. In C. Christiansen (Ed.), *Ways of Living*. Bethesda, MD: American Occupational Therapy Association.
Hemphill-Pearson, B. (1999). *Assessments in occupational therapy mental health*. Thorofare, NJ: Slack.
Hettler, W. (1990). Wellness: The lifetime goal of a university experience. In J.D. Matarazzo (Ed.), *Behavioral health: A handbook of health enhancement and disease prevention*. New York: John Wiley and Sons.
Hoff, B. (1982). *The tao of pooh*. New York: Dutton.
Jackson, J. (1999). The Well Elderly Study. Workshop sponsored by the American Occupational Therapy Association. Philadelphia, PA.
Johnson, J. (1986). *Wellness: A context for living*. Thorofare, NJ: Slack.
Johnson, J. (1993). Wellness programs. In H. Hopkins & H. Smith (Eds.), *Willard and Spackman's occupational therapy* (8th ed). Lippincott: Philadelphia.
Kalat, J. (1998). *Biological psychology*. Brooks Cole Publishing: Pacific Grove, CA.
Kielhofner, G. & Burke, J. (1983). The evolution of knowledge and practice in occupational therapy: Past, present and future. In G. Kielhofner (Ed.) *Health through occupation*. Philadelphia: F.A. Davis.
Law, M. (Ed.) (1998). *Client centered occupational therapy*. Thorofare, NJ: Slack.
Law, M., Baptiste, S., McColl, M., Opzoomer, A., Palatajko, H. & Pollock, N. (1990). The Canadian Occupational Performance Measure: An outcome measure for occupational therapy. *Canadian Journal of Occupational Therapy*, 57, pp. 82-87.
Marcus, J. (1999). *Community health: Education and promotion manual*. Gaithersburg, MD: Aspen Publications.
Mattingly, C. & Fleming, M. (1993). *Clinical reasoning: Forms of inquiry in therapeutic practice*. Philadelphia: F.A. Davis.
Meyer, A. (1922). The philosophy of occupation therapy. *Archives of Occupational Therapy, 1:1*.
Moyers, B. (1993). *Healing and the mind*. New York: Doubleday.
Moyers, P. (1999). The guide to occupational therapy practice. *American Journal of Occupational Therapy*, 53(3): pp. 251-322.
Moyers, P. (2000). Integrating uniform terminology into practice. Workshop sponsored by the American Occupational Therapy Association. Hartford, CT, June 15.
Neistadt, M. & Crepeau, E. (1998). *Willard and Spackman's occupational therapy* (9th ed). Philadelphia, PA: Lippincott.
Opatz, J.P. (1985). A primer of health promotion. Washington, DC: Oryn Publishers.
Pauls, J. & Reed, K. (1996). *Quick reference to physical therapy*. Gaithersburg, MD: Aspen Publications.
Pert, C. (1997). *Molecules of emotion*. New York: Scribner.

Pizzi, M. (1996). HIV and wellness strategies. *OT Week*, January, 25, pp. 17-18.

Pizzi, M. (1997). *Wellness Assessment and Intervention Strategies*. Paper presented at the National Geriatric Wellness and Rehabilitation Conference, Tampa, FL.

Pizzi, M. (1998). *The Holistic Wellness Assessment*. National Center for Wellness and Health Promotion: Silver Spring, MD.

Reed, K.L. (1991). *Quick reference to occupational therapy*. Gaithersburg, MD: Aspen Publications.

Reed, K. & Sanderson, S. (1999). *Concepts of occupational therapy, 4th Edition*. Philadelphia, PA: Lippincott.

Reilly, M. (1962). Occupational therapy can be one of the great ideas of the 20th century. *American Journal of Occupational Therapy*, 16, pp. 1-9.

Reilly, M. (1969). The educational process. *American Journal of Occupational Therapy*, *23*, p. 299.

Ryan, R.S. & Travis, J.W. (1991). *Wellness: Small changes you can use to make a big difference*. Berkeley, CA: Ten Speed Press.

Slagle, E.C. (1922). Training aides for mental patients. *Archives of Occupational Therapy*, *1:1*.

Van Deusen, J. & Brunt, D. (1997*). Assessment in occupational therapy and physical therapy*. Philadelphia, PA: Saunders.

von Bertalanffy, L. (1968). *General systems theory*. New York: George Braziller.

Weil, A. (1995). *Spontaneous healing*. New York: Knopf.

West, W. (1967). Professional responsibility in times of change. In *A professional legacy: The Eleanor Clarke Slagle lectures in occupational therapy 1955-1984*. American Occupational Therapy Association: Rockville, MD, 175-189.

Zemke, R. & Clark, F. (1996). *Occupational science: The evolving discipline*. F.A. Davis: Philadelphia.

Gateway to Wellness:
An Occupational Therapy Collaboration
with the National Multiple Sclerosis Society

Peggy Neufeld, MA, OTR/L
Kathy Kniepmann, MPH, EdM, CHES, OTR/L

SUMMARY. Occupational therapy is well equipped to build wellness for people with disabilities, particularly when partnering with community agencies or organizations. This article describes the collaborative relationship with the National Multiple Sclerosis Society for the development of Gateway to Wellness, A Program for Individuals with Multiple Sclerosis. Using the metaphor of a journey, issues relating to the collaborative relationship include language and power, paths and directions, the model design and evaluation, and negotiating expansion. The authors conclude with a summary of recommendations for positive part-

---

Peggy Neufeld, doctoral candidate, is Instructor in the Program of Occupational Therapy at the Washington University School of Medicine, 4444 Forest Park Boulevard, St. Louis, MO 63108. Kathy Kniepmann is Instructor and Coordinator of Student Activities, Program in Occupational Therapy, Washington University School of Medicine.

The authors thank their partners from the National Multiple Sclerosis Society, in particular Cindy Sorensen, Pat Knoerle-Jordan, Deborah Hertz, Cindee McLaughlin, and Deborah Frankel.

The Gateway to Wellness project was supported in part by grants from the Education and Training Foundation, Spinal Cord Injury, Paralyzed Veterans of America, 1997 to 1999, and the Gateway Area Chapter, National Multiple Sclerosis Society, 1997 to 2000.

nering between occupational therapy and organizations that serve persons with disabling conditions. *[Article copies available for a fee from The Haworth Document Delivery Service: 1-800-342-9678. E-mail address: <getinfo@haworthpressinc.com> Website: <http://www.HaworthPress.com> © 2001 by The Haworth Press, Inc. All rights reserved.]*

KEYWORDS. Collaboration, community health, empowerment, health promotion, multiple sclerosis

The Gateway to Wellness Program for persons with multiple sclerosis began with a phone call from the local chapter of the National Multiple Sclerosis Society. They were looking for a speaker on energy conservation. As an occupational therapy faculty member, I often receive such requests to present in the community. But the discussion that followed became the jumping point for developing a community program. I asked about other programs the chapter offered and realized that they offered few fitness and health education programs. When I described a fitness program that my occupational therapy program offered for persons with Parkinson's Disease, the chapter person was excited about a similar possibility for persons with multiple sclerosis (MS). This was the beginning of a collaborative journey that would establish wellness programs for people with MS across the nation. (Peggy Neufeld)

This article continues this story to describe how such requests can be explored for expansion beyond a single presentation to become sustained contributions to wellness and occupational performance for populations with disabling conditions. Health and wellness programs have gained considerable attention for their potential benefits to the general population in terms of lifestyles, quality of life and economic benefits (Clayton, Rogers & Stuifbergen, 1999; Gold, 2000; U.S. Department of Health and Human Services, 1991; Watt, Verma & Flynn, 1998). People with chronic disease and disabling conditions represent an increasing proportion within the general US population (Parrino, 2000). Because of their health conditions and/or impairments, they may require wellness programs that are tailored for persons with particular occupational performance challenges (DeJong, 1995; Gold, 2000; Kniepmann, 1997; Marge, 1988; Patrick, 1997; Patrick, Richardson, Starks, Rose, & Kinne, 1997; Rimmer, 1999; Stuifbergen & Rogers,

1997). As the need for health and wellness programs is recognized for people with disabling conditions, questions emerge: "How should wellness be defined and promoted?" and "Who should provide wellness programs?"

In the health and medical fields, universal definitions of wellness do not currently exist. The term wellness overlaps with concepts of health and health promotion, and at times they are used interchangeably. Christiansen (1999) makes the distinction that being healthy is different from being well and that "health enables people to pursue the tasks of everyday living that provide them with the life meaning necessary for their well-being" (p. 547). This distinction appears consistent with Stuifbergen's (1997) description of health promoting behaviors as essential for increasing levels of well-being. In her study, interviews with persons with MS expanded typical descriptions of health promoting behaviors beyond good habits of sleep, nutrition, and exercise to include maintaining a positive attitude, seeking and receiving interpersonal support and lifestyle adjustment.

These concepts of health and health promotion are closely related to that of wellness. On the other hand, wellness has a broader range of definitions. Wellness has been defined as a dynamic integration of mind, body, spirit, emotions and environment (Johnson, 1986) or as proactive health behaviors (Reitz, 1992). Others define wellness as choosing personally meaningful occupations for a self-identified balance in one's lifestyle (Jackson, Carlson, Mandel, Zembke & Clarke, 1998), or as an active process of becoming aware of and making choices toward a personally satisfying lifestyle (Carness, 1998). For the purpose of this paper, wellness is considered an individually defined attitude that empowers active pursuit of a balance of occupations (self-care, leisure, and productivity) to satisfy the preferences and needs of the mind, body, emotions, spirit and environment. Furthermore, having a wellness attitude or "mind-set" encourages routine participation in health promoting behaviors.

Occupational Therapy (OT) is well equipped to build wellness programs, particularly when partnering with community agencies or organizations. Baum and Law (1998) charge occupational therapists to collaborate with communities and organizations to build programs that enable a sense of wellness and a positive quality of life in persons with chronic disease. Rosenfeld (1993) affirms that OT can offer more than symptomatic treatment as he elegantly outlines the potential results of an OT wellness and lifestyle renewal program. In further support of the role of OT in community wellness programming, Fearing, Law and

Clark (1997) declare, "the art of occupational therapy includes the ability to create healthy environments where clients can grow and change while remaining firmly grounded within the context of their own lives" (p. 12).

Partnering can be the vehicle that enables stronger and more sustained wellness programs. This requires awareness of the less visible aspects of collaboration that may hinder the process. One means of paving the way for mutual growth and innovative, meaningful wellness programs is through reflection and critical analysis of the more hidden realities of collaboration.

Using the metaphor of a journey, this paper describes a model of occupational therapy collaboration with the National Multiple Sclerosis Society (NMSS) to provide wellness programs for persons with MS. In any journey, the traveler carves out opportunities and chooses paths or directions. The journey becomes a joint construction or collaboration with those met along the way. The reality of a collaborative journey is a range of possible interactions, from an agreeable partnering to a clash of conflicting agendas. This paper discusses issues related to collaborating in community practice, describes the development and current status of the Gateway to Wellness program, and concludes with a summary of suggestions for occupational therapists to consider when partnering with organizations serving individuals with disabilities.

RECOGNIZING ISSUES OF LANGUAGE AND POWER IN A COLLABORATIVE JOURNEY

What does collaboration really look like? The term collaboration is typically described with words such as agreement, sharing, and partnership. These terms reflect that collaboration provides important opportunities for building on complementary interests and goals. On the other hand, everyday language also refers to collaboration using words such as conflict, resistance, and negotiation. These latter terms show the hidden realities of collaboration. Recognizing these hidden realities is an important step to building strategies for successful collaboration. Allowing differences to be understood or overcome brings complementary interests to the forefront in collaboration.

Examining definitions of collaboration from an education and research perspective may be a useful place to begin clarifying this concept. Clark et al. (1996) describe collaboration as "not doing the same work, but rather, in terms of understanding the work of one another"

(p. 196). Buber (as cited in John-Steiner, Weber, & Miniis, 1998) adds another dimension to the definition by stating that collaboration is "more than the sum of individual participants; there is shared knowledge of an *emergent form*" (p. 775). In other words, the collaborative process cannot be reduced to the separate knowledge of the individuals, but is new knowledge constructed in a joint fashion.

These definitions suggest that ways of talking (dialogue among participants) are the centerpiece of collaborative exchange. Within dialogue, language serves as a cultural tool to mediate meanings and enable or constrain subsequent understanding and collaboration (Wertsch, 1991, 1998). Language is laden with multiple meanings–meanings that each participant brings from his or her different contexts and different points of view. Thus, language is not neutral. This perspective highlights that collaboration is more than a simple process of transferring and joining information. Participants must negotiate and jointly construct meanings over time, with language serving to shape new ways of knowing (knowledge) or levels of understanding. During negotiation the collaborators position themselves and others in relationships of power. Collaboration then becomes a process of aligning and realigning power through ways of talking and ways of knowing.

An important feature of language and power in collaboration is that participants are frequently unaware of the ways language realigns power. The dialogue in a collaborative process often remains unexamined. As a framework to understand collaborative efforts, it is important to recognize that positive partnering results from an ongoing examination of the dialogic points of difference and possible tension. These points become critical moments in which collaborative efforts can change. For example, during the collaborative work of building a wellness program for persons with multiple sclerosis, participants initially assumed that each shared similar meanings of the words "wellness" and "health education." In reality, the collaborators (in this case occupational therapists who were also university faculty members, and the managers of a national disability organization who came from different disciplinary backgrounds) brought multiple meanings to the discussion–meanings based on their theoretical perspectives and prior contexts.

During the collaborative journey of building a national wellness program for persons with MS, a number of given differences and points of tension emerged. For example, collaborators brought cultural and language differences based on the structures and particular working methods of their institutions. The use of language specific to professional disciplines sometimes brought miscommunication and related territoriality issues. Institutional differences raised issues of ownership for the new project. Basic beliefs about education and research needed to be examined. Throughout the shared work, meanings had to be constructed about the definition of wellness. Ongoing discussion was necessary to describe the appearance of a national wellness program. Throughout the collaborative journey, participants fluctuated in awareness of these points but came to realize that examination and clarification of points of difference paved the way for positive partnering.

CHOOSING PATHS AND PARTNERS

Establishing the wellness program required numerous actions at the local level before national connections were made. After the initial telephone conversation between the occupational therapist and the staff from the Gateway Area Chapter of the NMSS, a needs assessment identified concerns and perspectives from persons with MS, health professionals, the NMSS and its local chapter, and related research literature. What types of programs had the chapter offered before and what is offered currently? How were the current and past education and wellness programs viewed by persons with MS and the chapter? What occupational performance areas are threatened by the symptoms of MS? What education models for wellness demonstrate efficacy in improved quality of life for persons with MS or related chronic disease?

The needs assessment found the Gateway Area Chapter of the NMSS ready to support new wellness programs for its members. The Chapter had recently offered an exercise course led by a physical therapist, but with limited attendance. Investigation into that program revealed important considerations for future programming. For example, the exercise course was offered in late afternoons on hospital grounds. This site and schedule suited the hospital-based therapist's schedule for least conflict with revenue producing work time. However, persons experiencing MS fatigue found it difficult to attend partly due to the time of day (late afternoon) and the location (a long walk from parking). Additionally, the hospital location promoted an image of illness, not wellness, an important issue for persons with chronic disabling conditions.

Specific conditions related to MS needed to be considered during programming. Neurological symptoms of MS are varied and the course of the disease is variable and unpredictable. No cure is available and multiple symptoms interfere with physical and psychosocial functioning. The majority of individuals diagnosed with MS are women (3 out of 4), with the onset during the 20s or 30s. Thus, women are occupationally challenged in many life activities of career development, parenting, and/or finding a life partner or spouse.

Consultation with health professionals who work with persons with MS revealed differences in basic beliefs about wellness education. Some felt that a disease-specific education program (solely for persons with MS) should segregate participants based on physical abilities, such as a program designated only for wheelchair users. Those health professionals felt that persons who were newly diagnosed or "minimally disabled" should not be placed in a program with others in wheelchairs because it would be too depressing. This assumes that ambulation is a criterion of function and disability, which is questionable. Furthermore, such segregation places obstacles to inclusion in community programs. Beliefs also differed in desired program outcomes. Some health professionals felt that wellness program outcomes should focus on specific exercise benefits of strength and joint flexibility; others supported outcomes at the level of improved perception and confidence of exercise capacity and lifestyle routines.

To include the voices of persons with MS and their family members in the needs assessment, opinions were gathered with a telephone interview of twenty-five people. The local chapter of the NMSS announced the interview opportunity in their newsletter. Phone interviews identified possible content (priority topics), educational process (learning activities), and logistics (preferred scheduling and location, and transportation needs). The interest in a wellness program was overwhelmingly positive and interviewees spoke of a wide range of occupational challenges. Of the predominantly middle-aged survey respondents, fifty percent needed classes during day hours and the others who still worked needed after-work scheduling.

Building on studies of programs using models of empowerment, health promotion and wellness (Anderson et al., 1995; Braden, McGlone, & Pennington, 1993; Lorig & Holman, 1993; Lorig et al., 1999; Rappaport, 1984), a new wellness program was conceptualized for persons with MS. Broadly speaking, empowerment refers to an individual's capacity to use personal, social, or political power to create change (Bernstein et al., 1994). Beyond controlling personal capacities and the environment, empowerment includes ways of thinking about the environment (Wallerstein & Bernstein, 1988). Using this perspective, the developing wellness program encouraged participatory learning and an active, cooperative and dialogic process (Freire, 1985; Shor, 1992). The aim of empowerment was further enhanced through application of Bandura's (1986) Social Learning Theory with its emphasis on facilitating self-efficacy (confidence for performing specific tasks) through role modeling and mastery experiences. Additionally, drawing on the Person-Environment-Occupation (PEO) Model and its focus on occupational performance as the interaction of PEO factors in everyday activities (Baum & Law, 1997; Law et al., 1996), the wellness program facilitated empowerment through encouraging group members to recognize themselves as experts bringing personal knowledge from experiences in everyday activities.

The developing wellness program benefited from a growing body of literature on self-management of the consequences of chronic disease (Clark et al., 1991; Holman & Lorig, 1992). In particular, research from Lorig and her colleagues (1993) document the dramatic effects of gaining self-efficacy for self-management skills. Lorig and colleagues found that self-efficacy for self-management skills (and not simply knowledge) mediated lifestyle changes and psychosocial adjustments in persons with arthritis–resulting in the participant's experience of pain decreasing and number of hospitalizations reducing (Lorig & Holman, 1993; Lorig et al., 1999). Critical self-management skills for chronic health conditions as described by Holman and Lorig (1992) are:

- Gaining and maintaining physical fitness to avoid physical deconditioning
- Setting realistic expectations and emotional adjustments for self
- Interpreting and managing disease symptoms
- Managing the effects of medications
- Problem solving for fluctuations of daily abilities or environmental conditions
- Communicating with health professionals in partnerships
- Finding and using community resources

THE GATEWAY TO WELLNESS MODEL

Design and objectives. The current Gateway to Wellness program for individuals with multiple sclerosis evolved from a course that was offered twice a year from 1993 to 1997. The six-week program of education, exercise, and goal setting is comprised of once a week sessions. Each two-hour session includes discussion on two topics (thirty minutes each), a thirty-minute exercise session, and ends with goal setting. Each person sets a personal goal for the following week and discusses progress toward the past week's goals. The programs are offered at community sites that meet space and accessibility requirements. Ten to fifteen participants attend a program and each pays a nominal registration fee. The general objectives for Gateway to Wellness are for participants to:

1. Demonstrate skills to manage the consequences of MS.
2. Demonstrate confidence in skills to manage the consequences of MS.
3. Identify options and adopt a healthy lifestyle.
4. Build networks with individuals and community agencies for continued support and education.

Leadership. Because this is an empowerment-based program, the leader is not viewed as the expert who has all the answers. Rather, group members are encouraged to see themselves as experts bringing authentic everyday knowledge from their personal experiences. Group members learn from the wisdom of all the participants, not just from the program leader, as they share in problem solving the challenges of living with MS. Knowledge, skills, and attitude changes come from each participant actively "teaching" (informally through sharing experiences and perspectives) and learning (or listening and trying out new ideas) from everyone in the group. All participants, as well as the leaders, function as teachers and learners. Each uses the Gateway to Wellness experiences in ways that are meaningful for his or her own life. To become a leader for Gateway to Wellness, disciplinary knowledge is less critical than knowing how to facilitate empowering learning environments. A variety of health professionals, including the occupational therapist or therapy assistant, physical therapist or therapy assistant, social worker, nurse, or a therapeutic recreation specialist, have been trained to become Gateway to Wellness leaders. The criterion that the leader must be a health professional assumes shared core beliefs about health practices. Most importantly, leaders are trained at a Leader Training Program for Gateway to Wellness, administered by the NMSS (Neufeld, 1999a; Neufeld & Kniepmann, 2000).

During a Leader Training Program co-leaders and chapter staff managers are also trained in the Gateway to Wellness philosophy and strategies. The working team of a leader, co-leader, and chapter staff contributes to the success of this community education model. Active involvement of a co-leader who is diagnosed with MS emphasizes the empowering way of learning through role modeling. Sharing personal experience with others with chronic disease has a persuasive power for learning self-management confidence and skills. The third team member is a chapter staff member of NMSS who manages the program. Managing Gateway to Wellness includes marketing the program, coordinating leaders for local scheduling, recruiting and registering participants, and monitoring program evaluations.

Content. Sessions address occupations of self-care, play, and productivity, adapting home and work environments, and maintaining roles such as spouse/partner, parent, employed worker and volunteer. Discussions include coping with fatigue, cognitive or other physical symptoms and managing emotional and social changes. Communication skills are emphasized to enable participant partnering with family, friends, organizations and health professionals in the journey toward wellness. A hands-on unit exploring the computer and the Internet Super Highway points our wellness benefits from going on-line. Weekly "homework pages" are provided as one way to foster personal reflection on needs and interests and help participants prepare for each session (Neufeld, 1999b). Participants decide whether (or how much) to do these assignments based on their own interests. Decisions to share are left with each group member. In each session, the co-leaders outline a problem or question and encourage dialogue and problem solving. Such methods are consistent with social learning theory and the empowerment model. Sharing personal stories is also encouraged as a way of knowing or knowledge (Bruner, 1986). Story telling may be helpful in making meaning of illness experiences and promoting future stories of healthy adapting and coping. The final session is a celebration by the group as each member is recognized for his or her participation and members identify goals or plans for continued work in the following weeks.

Weekly physical exercises are chosen based on their potential to increase and maintain flexibility and endurance. The leader routinely reviews guidelines about when and how to modify the exercises and activities in order for group members to learn safe exercise practices. Specific types of exercises vary from floor or chair routines to Tai Chi, Yoga, or parachute and game activities. An important goal of the weekly exercise sessions is to promote each participant's learning how to adapt exercises to individual needs, how to monitor fatigue and safety during exercising, and how to build exercise into lifestyle routines.

In the final thirty minutes of each session, personal goal setting serves as a powerful means to support each group member's confidence in and application of self-management skills in his or her daily life. The program leaders guide group members to set specific measurable goals that are achievable in the following week. Each week, participants report to the group about their performance and set new goals as desired. Individual goals range from exercise routines, to accommodating work or home environments for better fit, to taking specific social or educational initiatives.

Criteria for enrollment. The criteria for enrolling in Gateway to Wellness include having a diagnosis of MS or being a partner of a person with MS. Some chapters require a doctor verification of the diagnosis. Group members must be able to participate in the exercises with no more than minimal assistance from the leader, take part in individual reflection assignments, and contribute to group skills training and discussions without interfering with other group members' learning. There are no criteria regarding specific disability levels. This allows group members with "invisible" symptoms such as fatigue, sensory or cognitive loss, to participate along with those with observable difficulties such as ambulation requiring wheelchair or ambulatory aids. To prepare group members for the program and to ensure retention in the program, the Gateway to Wellness manager informs group members upon their registration that other group members could represent a wide range of possible MS-related abilities and experiences.

Program evaluation. The initial wellness courses were a pilot community program and evaluation model. Faculty could explore research questions and occupational therapy students could learn about community models while assisting in the field. Program evaluations were positive during the first four years when Neufeld and Kniepmann offered the wellness courses in St. Louis, Missouri. Positive outcomes were documented through participants' high ratings on achieving personal goals, satisfaction with the program, increased confidence in using self-management skills for the consequences of MS and testimonials on adaptive changes in daily living activities. The local chapter of NMSS requested additional programs. This required leader training so others could offer this well-received community program to a larger population.

NEGOTIATING EXPANSION

New administrative and funding partners. Finding a funding partner for expansion of the wellness program was a challenge. Early proposals for funding directed at local and national organizations were unsuccessful, including early requests to the National Multiple Sclerosis Society. The Education and Training Foundation of the Paralyzed Veterans of America (ETF/PVA) was identified as a potential funding source. PVA was interested in programming for persons with MS because a large percent of their membership had spinal cord dysfunction due to MS. ETF of PVA was interested in training programs, manuals, and program evaluations. The turning point for expansion of the wellness program came when ETF/PVA provided a substantial two-year grant. Funding in the first year supported development of a Leader's Manual, Participant's Workbook and a leader training program; the second year supported the evaluation of the new wellness programs.

The Gateway Area Chapter of the NMSS, the local partners in St. Louis, matched the PVA grant. The additional funds supported the national office of the NMSS to plan and implement a three-year rollout of further leader training programs for wellness courses throughout the United States. The course was renamed "Gateway to Wellness, A Program for Individuals with MS," and the NMSS administered the program nationally.

While the national office of the NMSS adopted Gateway to Wellness as their self-management program, their "buy in" to the program was gradual. Staff explained that decisions are made cautiously in the organization's administrative structure and that the program developer was viewed as an "outsider." This appeared to cause confusion because an "outsider" to the NMSS developed the program and requested partnering. As the NMSS viewed the first drafts of the written Leader's Manual and the Participant's Workbook, some differences and tension came to the forefront. Just who had ownership of the program? Would the author be flexible in writing the manuals in order to be consistent with the NMSS philosophy?

Differences in educational philosophy and styles became apparent as the NMSS suggested downplaying or dropping theoretical foundations and urged a bulleted "how to" style for the manuals. Multiple conference calls with key players revealed distinct language differences among the partners. The author of the Gateway to Wellness manuals was an occupational therapist and faculty member operating from an empowerment, wellness model and accustomed to academic freedom without mandates on publication style or educational approaches. Working with the national organization required attention to other institutional ways of operating. The NMSS was an organization with a strong emphasis on medical expertise and viewpoints, operating from a medical model orientation, although highly interested in embracing a wellness model. In addition, their staff represented a wide variety of health professionals with differing disciplinary beliefs. Questions by the NMSS personnel during planning and training included, How should a national program look? What is wellness? Did this new program promote a concept of wellness that the NMSS advocated? What commitments would be required of the local chapters who sent personnel to the leader training program?

Evaluating outcomes. The collaboration of the ETF/PVA and the NMSS with the program developer made it possible for research to occur concurrently with training on the national level. The regionally trained teams of Gateway to Wellness leader, co-leader and chapter staff agreed to collect data from the participants of their first programs. Evaluation of the new leaders at post-training indicated satisfaction with their training program. After the new Gateway to Wellness programs were offered, leaders reported teaching the program in a manner consistent with their training. Program evaluations from the participants with MS and their partners indicated satisfaction with the Gateway to Wellness program. Group members particularly liked the combination of discussion with others with MS, exercise at each session, the access to information, the leader and co-leader model, the goal setting and the workbook. The most frequent complaint was that the program was too short or ended too soon.

An outcome study for the program collected data using pre- and post-program written questionnaires including demographics and a self-report on the Expanded Disability Status Scale (Solari, 1993). The outcome measures included participant rating of achievement of personal goals for attending the program, a measure on perceived knowledge relating to the program topics and developed for this study, quality of life assessments including the SF36 Health Status Survey (Ware & Sherbourne, 1992) and the Fatigue Severity Scale (Krupp, LaRocca & Muir-Nash, 1989), an assessment of self-efficacy for self-management of the consequences of MS (a modification of Lorig et al., 1989), and a report of frequency of use of self-management behaviors (Lorig, Stewart, Ritter, Laurent & Lynch, 1996).

The outcome study currently in progress is documenting positive trends (Neufeld, 1999c). For example, over a six-month period in 1998, 88% of the 149 participants (131) who were enrolled in 14 programs across the nation completed at least four of the six sessions. The participant's mean age is 48 years and their mean self-reported Expanded Disability Status Score of 4.6 indicates a substantial level of disability (walking limited distances and some other neurological symptoms).

The positive outcomes indicated include a majority of participants achieving personal goals at the completion of the program. Statistically significant changes included decreased fatigue interfering with daily activities (as measured on the Fatigue Severity Scale), increased perceived knowledge on program topics (e.g., community resources and therapy options for MS, stress and energy management), increased self-efficacy for self-management behaviors, and increased frequency in selected self-management behaviors (e.g., frequency of weekly exercise, attendance to support groups or classes about health, and use of methods to help memory).

THE JOURNEY CONTINUES AND RECOMMENDATIONS FOR POSITIVE PARTNERING

Upon reflecting on this ongoing journey for Gateway to Wellness, the authors suggest a number of actions for positive partnering:

- First, connect with a community agency(s) early in the planning process and invite them to dialogue. Create opportunities for multiple voices to begin clarifying interests and differences.
- Second, recognize and offer your unique OT knowledge, skills, and philosophy to the project. This stance will open doors for personal and professional change and growth.
- Third, approach differences as pivotal points for positive change, not as obstacles. Take time to actively listen to new partners. Reflect on and analyze the interactions to promote further dialogue over differences.
- Fourth, identify cultural differences in language that reflect differences in thinking (or knowing) and in beliefs. Learn about the partner's organizing schemes, philosophies, mission, and current activities. Understanding differences in language and activities paves the way toward alternative directions and alternative ways of talking.
- Fifth, strive for mutual empowerment of collaborating partners. This requires identifying strategies and implementing them within an ongoing dialogue from everyone's perspectives. Voice is a central shared feature of collaboration and a stepping-stone to empowerment.
- Finally, build in methods to evaluate impacts and outcomes of new collaborative programs. Monitor changes and responses to new

programs that will address or answer the various perspectives of the partners. Documentation of outcomes provides important evidence for program success and opens possibilities for further partnerships.

This collaborative journey has been an exciting opportunity for personal and professional growth for the authors of this paper. Currently thirty chapters of the NMSS across the United States have trained personnel to implement Gateway to Wellness. The NMSS continues as the administrative and funding manager of the new and ongoing Gateway to Wellness programs. In addition, seven Master Trainer pairs were recently trained to provide more leader training programs at new chapter sites throughout the United States. Many more persons with MS will have the opportunity to participate in this program that promotes wellness while living with a potentially devastating disease. For information about the availability of a Gateway to Wellness program for persons with MS in your region, or if you are interested in training to become a leader, telephone 1-800-FIGHT-MS to speak to a staff member from your local chapter of the NMSS.

REFERENCES

Anderson, R.M., Funnell, M.M., Butler, P.M., Arnold, M.S., Fitzgerald, J.T., & Feste, C.C. (1995). Patient empowerment, results of a randomized controlled trial. *Diabetes Care, 18*, 943-949.

Bandura, A. (1986). *Social foundations of thought and action: A social cognitive theory.* Englewood Cliffs, NJ: Prentice-Hall.

Baum, C., & Law, M. (1997). Occupational therapy practice: Focusing on occupational performance. *American Journal of Occupational Therapy, 51*, 277-288.

Baum, C. & Law, M. (1998). Community health: A responsibility, an opportunity and a fit for occupational therapy. *American Journal of Occupational Therapy, 52*, 7-10.

Bernstein, E., Wallerstein, H., Braithwaite, R., Gutierrez, L., Labonte, R., & Zimmerman, M. (1994). Empowerment forum: A dialogue between guest editorial board members. *Health Education Quarterly, 21*, 281-294.

Braden, C.J., McGlone, K. & Pennington, F. (1993). Specific psychosocial and behavioral outcomes from the Systemic Lupus Erythematosus Self-Help Course. *Health Education Quarterly, 20*, 29-42.

Bruner, J. (1986). *Actual minds, Possible worlds.* Cambridge, MA: Harvard University Press.

Carness, F. (1998). A wellness approach to disease state management. *Wellness Management, 14*, 4-5.

Christiansen, C. (1999). Defining lives: Occupation as identity: An essay on competence, coherence, and the creation of meaning–the 1999 Eleanor Clarke Slagle Lecture. *American Journal of Occupational Therapy, 53,* 547-558.

Clark, C., Moss, P.A., Goering, S., Herter, R.J., Lamar, B., Leonard, D., Robbins, S.,
Russell, M., Templin, M., & Wascha, K. (1996). Collaboration as dialogue:
Teachers and researcher engaged in conversation and professional development.
American Educational Research Journal, 33, 193-231.

Clark, N.M., Becker, M.H., Janz, J.K., Lorig, K., Rakowski, W., & Anderson, L.
(1991). Self-management of chronic disease by older adults–A review and questions for research. *Journal of Aging and Health, 3,* 3-27.

Clayton, D.K., Rogers, S., & Stuifbergen, A. (1999). Answers to unasked questions:
Writing in the margins. *Research in Nursing & Health, 22,* 512-522.

Dejong, G. (1995). *Preventing and managing secondary conditions in an era of managed care.* Paper presented at the Conference on Secondary Conditions and Aging
with a Disability, Syracuse, NY.

Fearing, V.G., Law, M., & Clark, J. (1997). An occupational performance process
model: Fostering client and therapist alliances. *Canadian Journal of Occupational
Therapy, 64,* 7-15.

Freire, P. (1985). *The Politics of Education: Culture, power, and liberation,* translated
by P. Macedo. South Hadley, MA: Bergin & Garvey Publishers, Inc.

Gold, M. (2000). Healthy people 2000. In U. S. Department of Health and Human Services (Ed.), *National Conference on the Prevention of Primary and Secondary Disabilities: Healthy people 2010: National health promotion and disease prevention
objectives* (pp. 26-30). Washington, DC: U.S. Government Printing Office.

Holman, H., & Lorig, K. (1992). Perceived self-efficacy in self-management of
chronic disease. In R. Shwarzer (Ed.), *Self-Efficacy, Thought control of action*
(pp. 305-323). Washington, DC: Hemisphere Publishing Corp.

Jackson, J., Carlson, M., Mandel, D., Zembke, R. & Clark, F. (1998). Occupation in
lifestyle redesign: The well elderly study occupational therapy program. *American
Journal of Occupational Therapy, 42,* 326-336.

John-Steiner, V., Weber, R.J., & Miniis, M. (1998). The challenge of studying collaboration. *American Educational Research Journal, 35,* 773-783.

Johnson, J. (1986). Wellness and occupational therapy. *American Journal of Occupational Therapy, 40,* 753-758.

Kniepmann, K. (1997). Prevention of disability and maintenance of health. In C.
Christiansen & C. Baum (Eds.), *Occupational therapy: Enabling function and
well-being* (2nd edition), (pp. 530-555). Thorofare, NJ: SLACK Incorporated.

Krupp, L.B., LaRocca, N.G. & Muir-Nash, J. (1989). The fatigue severity scale: Application to patients with multiple sclerosis and systemic lupus erythematosus. *Archives of Neurology, 46,* 1121-23.

Law, M., Cooper, B.A., Strong, S., Stewart, D., Rigby, P., & Letts, L. (1996). The Per-
son-Environment-Occupational Model: A transactive approach to occupational
performance. *Canadian Journal of Occupational Therapy, 63,* 9-23.

Lorig, K., & Holman, M. (1993). Arthritis self-management studies: A twelve year review. *Health Education Quarterly, 20,* 17-28.

Lorig, K.R., Sobel, D.S., Stewart, A.L., Brown, B.W. Jr., Bandura, A., Ritter, P., Gonzalez, V.M., Laurent, D.D., & Holman, H.R. (1999). Evidence suggesting that a chronic disease self-management program can improve health status while reducing hospitalization: A randomized trial. *Medical Care, 37,* 5-14.

Lorig, K., Stewart, A., Ritter, P., Laurent, D., & Lynch, J. (1996). *Outcome measures for health education and other health care interventions.* Thousand Oaks, CA: Sage Publications.

Marge, M. (1988). Health promotion for people with disabilities: Moving beyond rehabilitation. *American Journal of Health Promotion, 2,* 29-44.

Neufeld, P. (1999a). *Leader's manual for Gateway to Wellness: A program for individuals with multiple sclerosis.* Denver, CO: National Multiple Sclerosis Society Training and Resource Center.

Neufeld, P. (1999b). *Participant's workbook for Gateway to Wellness: A program for individuals with multiple sclerosis.* Denver, CO: National Multiple Sclerosis Society Training and Resource Center.

Neufeld, P. (May, 1999c). *Promoting wellness in persons with MS.* A presentation in the Plenary Session of the Annual Conference of the Consortium of Multiple Sclerosis Societies. Kansas City, MO.

Neufeld, P. with Kniepmann, K. (2000). *Master training manual for Gateway to Wellness,* Denver, CO: National Multiple Sclerosis Society Training and Resource Center.

Parrino, S.S. (2000). National Council on Disability (NCD) historical perspective on prevention. In U.S. Department of Health and Human Services (Ed.), *National Conference on the Prevention of Primary and Secondary Disabilities: Healthy people 2010: National health promotion and disease prevention objectives* (pp. 15-20). Washington, DC: U.S. Government Printing Office.

Patrick, D. (1997). Rethinking prevention for people with disabilities part I: A conceptual model for promoting health. *American Journal of Health Promotion, 11,* 257-260.

Patrick, D., Richardson, M., Starks, H.E., Rose, M.A., & Kinne, S. (1997). Rethinking prevention for people with disabilities part II: A framework for designing interventions. *American Journal of Health Promotion, 11,* 261-263.

Rappaport, J. (1984). Studies in empowerment: Introduction to the issue. *Prevention in Human Services, 3,* 1-7.

Reitz, S.M. (1992). A historical review of occupational therapy's role in preventive health and wellness. *American Journal of Occupational Therapy, 46,* 50-55.

Rimmer, J.H. (1999). Health promotion for people with disabilities: The emerging paradigm shift from disability prevention to prevention of secondary conditions. *Physical Therapy, 79,* 495-502.

Rosenfeld, M. (1993). *Wellness and lifestyle renewal, A manual for personal change.* Rockville, MD: The American Occupational Therapy Association, Inc.

Shor, I. (1992). *Empowering education: Critical teaching for social change.* Chicago: The University of Chicago Press.

Solari, A., Amato, M., Bergamaschi, R., Logroscino, G., Citterio, A., Bochicchio, D., & Fillippini, G. (1993). Accuracy of self-assessment of the minimal record of disability in patients with multiple sclerosis. *Acta Neurologica Scandanavia, 87,* 43-46.

Stuifbergen, A.K., & Rogers, S. (1997). Health promotion: An essential component of rehabilitation for persons with chronic disabling conditions. *Advances in Nursing Science, 19,* 1-20.

U.S. Department of Health and Human Services. (1991). *National Conference on the Prevention of Primary and Secondary disabilities: Building partnerships towards health–Reducing the risks for disability.* Atlanta: Centers for Disease Control and Prevention.

Wallerstein, N., & Bernstein, E. (1988). Empowerment education: Freire's ideas adapted to health education. *Health Education Quarterly, 15,* 379-394.

Ware, J.E. & Sherbourne, C.D. (1992). The MOS 36-item Short Form Health Survey (SF036). *Medical Care, 30,* 473-481.

Watt, D., Verma, S., & Flynn, L. (1998). Wellness programs: A review of the evidence. *Canadian Medical Association Journal, 158,* 224-230.

Wertsch, J.V. (1998). *Mind as action.* New York: Oxford University Press.

Wertsch, J.V. (1991). *Voices of the mind.* Cambridge, MA: Harvard University.

Facilitating Successful International Adoptions: An Occupational Therapy Community Practice Innovation

Gale L. Haradon, PhD, OTR

SUMMARY. Occupational therapists are encouraged to enter community practice as international adoption consultants. Pre-adoption workshops on risks of institutionalization and family preparation are discussed. Assessment methods for evaluating records and videos are suggested. Post-adoption use of developmental examinations and information on common medical conditions of Russian and Romanian adoptees are discussed. *[Article copies available for a fee from The Haworth Document Delivery Service: 1-800-342-9678. E-mail address: <getinfo@haworthpressinc.com> Website: <http://www.HaworthPress.com> © 2001 by The Haworth Press, Inc. All rights reserved.]*

KEYWORDS. International, adoption, community, occupational therapy, developmental

---

Gale L. Haradon is Chair and Associate Professor, Department of Occupational Therapy, University of Texas Health Science Center, San Antonio. Address correspondence to: 7703 Floyd Curl Drive-6245, San Antonio, TX 78229-3900.

This article is dedicated with appreciation to the wonderful families and children the author has met during the past seven years who have allowed her to enter their lives during their exciting international adoption journeys.

[Haworth co-indexing entry note]: "Facilitating Successful International Adoptions: An Occupational Therapy Community Practice Innovation." Haradon, Gale L. Co-published simultaneously in *Occupational Therapy in Health Care* (The Haworth Press, Inc.) Vol. 13, No. 3/4, 2001, pp. 85-99; and: *Community Occupational Therapy Education and Practice* (eds: Beth P. Velde, and Peggy Prince Wittman) The Haworth Press, Inc., 2001, pp. 85-99. Single or multiple copies of this article are available for a fee from The Haworth Document Delivery Service [1-800-342-9678, 9:00 a.m. - 5:00 p.m. (EST). E-mail address: getinfo@haworthpressinc.com].

Extensive growth in the number of international adoptions has created a need for services from health professionals who are knowledgeable about international adoption and the effects of prior institutionalization on these children. Occupational therapists are ideally positioned to work with international adoption agencies, adoptive families and their children. Occupational therapists already are encountering international adoptees in familiar practice settings such as Early Childhood Intervention (ECI) programs, schools, and pediatric rehabilitation programs. Expanding these evaluation and intervention programs to include pre-adoption and post-adoption services to agencies and families is an appropriate community role. Increasing resources are now available for both health professionals and families to help in the understanding of the internationally adopted child (Ochs, 2000).

Institutionalized children are considered a high-risk group and parents are urged to become aware of the parenting challenges of this population and to prepare in advance of the adoption for the rehabilitation of their children (Johnson & Hostetter, 1999). Occupational therapists are educated to evaluate and work with children who exhibit special physical and mental health problems such as developmental delays, sensory integration deficits, behavioral problems, and feeding difficulties which are frequently present in the child who has been adopted from an international orphanage. The role of the occupational therapist in pre-adoption and post-adoption will be discussed in addition to background and research information that encompasses medical and developmental concerns common to this population.

The author has consulted for the past seven years with an international adoption agency. Her work has encompassed more than 30 workshop presentations to prospective parents and health professionals. She has reviewed "referral" medical and background information or performed developmental examinations on approximately 100 children adopted from Romanian and Russian orphanages. In addition to research studies that are presented from a variety of authors, her knowledge of the effects of institutionalization came from personal experience working with orphans for one year in Romania and consulting to health programs for one year in Romania and the Independent Republic of Moldova.

A guide to Russian diagnosis and medical terminology is found in a helpful reference called *Russian Children and Medical Records* (Jenista, 1997). Russian adoptions constitute the largest percentage of international adoptions to the United States. Other most represented countries with significant adoptions include China, Korea, Romania and South

American Countries. More than 40,000 children from institutions in Eastern Europe have been adopted in the United States since 1991 (Immigration & Naturalization Service, 1998). Many of the international adoptees are toddlers who have spent their first year(s) of life in an institution (Hopkins-Best, 1977).

The practice arena for consulting on international adoptions is ideally suited for experienced pediatric occupational therapists. A background in sensory integration and working with children with psychosocial problems is especially helpful when working with this population.

OCCUPATIONAL THERAPISTS' ROLE IN PRE-ADOPTION WORKSHOPS

Occupational therapists can become involved with an adoption agency by giving pre-adoption workshops and consulting at the time of a referral of a child to the family. The international adoption agency has an obligation to provide medical information about the child who is being placed with adoptive families and to help families make good decisions about the health issues that they are likely to encounter (Johnson & Hostetter, 1999; Merrill, 1996). Decisions that will affect adoptive families and children for the rest of their lives are best based upon unbiased information from health professionals and not solely on the basis of attractive photographs and videos (Merrill, 1996). Families are not obligated to accept a referral of a child from an adoption agency that they feel they are incapable of parenting.

Occupational therapists can aid in this information gathering by presenting workshops on the potential risks and benefits to families who are considering international adoption and by reviewing medical information and videos on the child when he/she is referred for the parents' adoption decision. The following workshop topics that are appropriate to present to families will be discussed:

- Risks of institutionalization (development, growth, feeding, attachment, sensory problems, central auditory processing and school readiness)
- Preparation and initial adjustment suggestions
- Post-adoption research
- Professional services and areas they address (occupational therapy, physical therapy, speech pathology, psychology, special education, early childhood intervention)
- Cultural data on child's country of origin

Risks of Institutionalization

Parents are encouraged to have their children evaluated by a physician after arrival in their new homes. In addition to the typical physical examination and immunizations, pediatricians need to evaluate for the presence of diseases that are commonly seen in this population. After the children have had two weeks to settle in to their new situations, they are encouraged to have a baseline developmental assessment. Johnson and Hostetter (1999) believe that most children over the age of two years need rehabilitation to correct deficits imposed from their orphanage life. Children may appear normal and later have problems such as attachment issues that show up after they are more secure in their new homes. Fine and gross motor delays are expected of all the children from their deprived backgrounds, but results have shown that a stimulating environment and nutrition cause children to catch up in these areas (Ames, Fisher, Morison, & Chisholm, 1999; Faber, 2000; Haradon, 1999a, b; Miller, 2000). Delays in language, social skills, behavioral problems and attachment may persist for a long time in some children (Federici, 1998; Johnson, 1999). The lack of stimulation during developing periods can lead to challenges in school, especially during transition periods from kindergarten to first grade where subtle learning disabilities and intellectual impairments surface. Johnson (1999) concluded after a review of 1000 institutionalized children that there is no way of predicting the needs of children adopted from orphanages since the situation changes with some earlier problems becoming resolved and other problems appearing with time. Children are invariably found to have impaired physical growth in an orphanage and lose one month of linear growth for every three months in an orphanage. Weight gain and head growth are also depressed (Johnson, 1999).

A group living situation fosters the spread of infectious agents, intestinal parasites, hepatitis B, tuberculosis, chicken pox and middle ear infections (Aronson, 2000; Crumpecker, 1977; Johnson, 1999, 2000). Children may also have been subjected to physical and/or sexual abuse in the orphanage in addition to poor nutrition, changing caregivers, and lack of stimulation for tactile, vestibular, auditory and emotional development.

Preparation and Initial Adjustment Suggestions

While parents seldom have the opportunity to gain insight from the orphanage staff on the life of the children at the orphanage, information on the customary day of the child prior to adoption is helpful to facilitate the child's adjustment to his/her new environment. Workshops can inform parents that the child has probably rarely been alone in a room, but has shared a room with approximately twenty-four other children who live in cribs or beds juxtaposed to one another. Undoubtedly the children have never taken a ride in an automobile prior to being picked up at the orphanage by the adopting parents. Possibly the child has spent his/her days in the confines of a single room or inside the orphanage without the opportunity to go outside or use playground equipment. The children are not accustomed to separate rooms for eating and sleeping and probably eat, play, and sleep in the same room. Separate bathrooms off the room are customary.

Life in the orphanage is very orderly with meals being delivered at scheduled times and strict limits put on behaviors. Having access to food in a home may lead to hoarding behavior, eating insatiably, or perhaps refusal to eat because of unfamiliar textures or food selections. Typically orphanage food is bland, and common fare in Romanian orphanages consists of soups, porridge, cheese, sausage and breads. The child in an orphanage becomes comfortable with limits and frequently will test limits severely upon adoption unless limits are clearly defined and consistently reinforced. In the orphanage, most caregivers are women, and children are not around men. Therefore, upon adoption, the child may react unpredictably to the father because of the unfamiliarity of the deeper voice and masculine mannerisms. If education is provided in international orphanages, their programs may emphasize rote memory of information and repetition and do not encourage free exploration such as is common in American pre-schools, where there are choices of play activities.

Suggestions to share with families, individually or through workshop formats, are to allow time for the child to adjust to the changes in his/her new world gradually by slowly introducing toys, visitors, trips, and activities to the child (Federici, 1998; Hopkins-Best, 1997; Merrill, 1996). Although difficult, efforts should be made to avoid overwhelming the child. Instead of allowing the child to choose from many options, suggest he/she choose from between two things at first. Parents are encouraged to set firm, realistic limits and to see each child as a unique personality with frequently strong wills.

Another expected adjustment is to become accustomed to continuity of caregivers since caregivers in the orphanage work on shifts and change several times daily. Changes in placement occur as the child grows within the orphanage. Sometimes adjustment problems occur because of the unfamiliar freedom and excitement that occurs in a home environment. In the orphanage, the child does not possess his/her own toys and may hoard new personal possessions or show lack of regard for possessions of others. Responses to frustrations may be tantrums and disagreeable behavior and a disregard for restrictions when testing new limits (Hopkins-Best, 1997).

Lack of emotional development from caregivers who share emotions with the child may also lead to the child having trouble showing correct emotions. She/he may smile when unhappy and appear to have a "mask" on her/his face. Parents can be urged to understand and share emotional responses with children and identify the child's feelings for them by saying they seem sad, angry, happy, etc., so the child can understand congruent behaviors.

Post-Adoption Research

A comprehensive study by Ames et al. (1999) followed 46 children who had been adopted from Romanian orphanages to families in Canada. Findings from this study demonstrated that 78% of the adopted children were delayed in all areas of motor and language development. Children were less delayed if they had been in the orphanage a shorter time, had experience with toys in the orphanage, were favorites of the caregivers and had been kept clean. After 4-1/2 years, the Romanian children had generally made great progress but most had not yet caught up with other children in the family. In regards to growth, 85% of the children were below the 10th percentile for weight when initially adopted; after 4-1/2 years, only 18% were below the 10th percentile for weight and 31% below the 10th percentile for height. The longer the children spent in the orphanage, the shorter they were for their age.

At the time of adoption 85% had medical problems, which consisted of intestinal parasites (31%), Hepatitis B (28%), and anemia (15%). By the age of 4-1/2, their health had greatly improved except for Hepatitis B. Problem behaviors at the time of adoption were eating problems (75%) such as refusing solid food and eating too much and stereotypical behaviors such as rocking and staring at moving hands and fingers (84%). Initial parental concerns were about medical and development but later on the most troublesome were behavioral, emotional and social issues (Ames et al., 1999).

Attachment is a common worry for parents considering international adoption. Bowlby (1958) found that children who are securely attached use parents as a secure base from which to explore the world and a place of refuge when distressed. Two-thirds of the orphans in the Ames et al.

study (1999) were able to attach to their new families, but one-third of them reported uncommon patterns of insecure attachment which related to indiscriminate friendliness (where they were persistent in overly friendly behavior with strangers). These researchers conjectured that being indiscriminately friendly in an orphanage was a tactic to get attention from caregivers. Other studies of internationally adopted children from institutions concluded that there was a close association between duration of deprivation and severity of attachment disorder behaviors (O'Connor & Rutter, 2000; Zeanah, 2000).

Other behavior problems noted in the Ames et al. study were eating voraciously, avoiding particular foods such as salads, lying quietly in bed without calling or trying to get up, employing stereotypical behaviors and withdrawal from other children. Initially children may be docile, quiet and passive, which may later drift to more aggressive behavior, overactivity and distractibility. Deficiency in peer relationships is sometimes problematic. However, some case studies show the resiliency of children, indicating their delays all but disappeared within the first year of adoption.

Professional Services

Ames et al. found that one-third of the parents in her study sought professional help, but with time, the problems declined or disappeared and the concerns of the parents changed. Parents of children adopted from Romania to Canada utilized the services of speech therapy, occupational therapy, infant development program and special needs daycare most often. Two-thirds of the families in this study of Romanian adoptees used at least one special service.

Information on development, activities for stimulating development, sensory problems, feeding behaviors, auditory processing and school readiness can be shared by occupational therapists. Symptoms that would be appropriate to refer a child to pediatric professionals would be of interest to parents of adopted children. Language development has been found to be most delayed and the most difficult to remediate following adoption (Haradon, 1999b). Referrals to speech pathologists who specialize in early development can be helpful since the child usually lacks the foundation of language development that is normally encouraged by parents during infancy (Day, 1982). When the child reaches school age, the early weak language foundation causes stress for the child as he/she is struggling with higher concepts. Special education resources and English as a second language are especially valuable resources. Early Childhood Intervention is helpful for families since many adopted children are under three years of age and need developmental stimulation.

Cultural Data on Child's Country of Origin

Information on the language, music, history, geography, food and ethnicity of the child's country of origin is helpful and interesting to parents who are adopting children from certain ethnic areas. Some support groups form according to country of origin while others relate simply to the fact that a child was internationally adopted. Slides and speakers who can display artifacts from the country can be arranged for workshops and seminars. The Romanian language is particularly unknown to prospective parents and common misconceptions can be corrected. The language of Romania is a romance language that is Latin based, contrary to the expectation based on the geographical placement of the country. Romanian is most similar to Italian but does contain Turkish words from the time of the Turkish occupations. Romania is a land rich in natural resources, located near the Black Sea and dotted with castles throughout the country. Such information about other countries of origin of international adoptees can be researched and shared with parents and children.

REVIEWING REFERRAL INFORMATION
(RECORDS AND VIDEOS)

Occupational therapists can develop new community roles helping prospective adoptive parents assess the developmental risks of adopting a specific child. Occupational therapists are encouraged to work collaboratively with physicians who are willing to be consulted by pre-adoptive families to interpret medical tests and illnesses with which the occupational therapist does not have expertise. Pre-adoptive parents are encouraged, and sometimes required by adoption agencies, to obtain a health professional's opinion before adopting a child from an international orphanage to enable the families to have a better understanding and assessment of the nature of the child's risks for development and medical conditions.

The process of completing the home study and required forms is a lengthy process that could take over a year for adopting parents to complete. When a child is available in the country of choice that approximates a match of the characteristics of gender and age that the family has specified, the process is known as a "referral" (Merrill, 1996). Information from the country is typically sparse and consists of family medical history, circumstances surrounding the pregnancy, labor and delivery, weight, length and head circumference at birth and at the time of referral. Developmental milestones may be included in addition to immunization records and health history. The information should be provided in English, but the information is usually incomplete and may be incorrect. Specific diagnoses are suspect and may be interpreted very differently from the same diagnoses in the United States. The occupational therapist can contribute to the interpretation of these records.

Jenista (2000) states that all Russian medical records contain neurologic diagnoses that are almost impossible to interpret because of the use of terms such as perinatal encephalopathy, hyperexcitability syndrome, spastic tetraparesis and pyramidal insufficiency which may be used to represent conditions that differ from the American interpretation of the diagnosis and may not be congruent with the accompanying videotapes of the children. The videotapes serve to confirm or refute the information that is contained in the medical record. The occupational therapist may assess the child's developmental level as mild or moderately delayed with no visible evidence of neurological involvement.

Jenista (2000) uses a risk assessment scale that explains the risks for what is known and not known about a prospective child and assesses the child as low risk, moderate risk or high risk. A low risk assessment based on review of the medical information and the videotape would be defined as no worrisome data present. Janista found that only 9% of Eastern European or Russian records were classified as low risk versus 37% from the rest of the world. "Moderate risk" was defined as having one or more factors likely to impact future functioning, such as moderate growth or developmental delay, an involuntary termination of parental rights, being small for gestational age, or known correctable conditions such as a ventricular septal defect.

"High risk" was defined as a known diagnosis of fetal alcohol syndrome or other irreparable problems such as premature delivery at less than 30 weeks, birth weight less than 1000 gm or severe growth or developmental retardation. The occupational therapist's role is to outline what is known and not known about a child and to estimate the resources the child might be expected to need with certain conditions. For example, if a child has a known condition which will need the resources of occupational and physical therapy, the cost and duration of treatment could be outlined to parents.

The occupational therapist is not expected to select a child for the parents. The role of reviewing the medical history, the photographs, and the videotape is to determine what is known, to generate questions to ask of orphanage personnel about the child and to determine medical specialists that need further consultation prior to making a pre-adoptive decision. This author finds it most beneficial to review the medical history and developmental history first and to make a mental image of this child in terms of health and condition. Then a review of the videotape can confirm the risks, disconfirm the report, or generate new questions to ask and issues to clarify. The author's experience as an occupational therapist reviewing records from Romania and Russia has shown a tremendous disparity of styles and completeness from different adoption contacts. An objective and supportive attitude is essential to develop a trusting relationship with the parent so the occupational therapist is not seen as persuading the parent to either accept or reject a particular referral or as connected with the adoption agency who has given the parent the referral.

The role of the occupational therapists is to clarify the risks and to support the parents in whatever decision they feel is best for their family. Since a false expectation can lead to negative consequences for a child's life and that of the adoptive family, acceptance of a child should never be made from a sense of guilt or being pressured to make a decision.

OCCUPATIONAL THERAPISTS' ROLE IN POST-ADOPTION

Occupational therapists can become involved with the adoption agency or family by administering appropriate assessments such as developmental and sensory integration evaluations. Community referrals, consultations, and support group seminars on topics of relevance to the new families are appropriate following adoption.

Assessments and Intervention

Medical conditions that are commonly seen in international adoptees (Aronson, 2000) include chronic upper respiratory or ear infections, diarrhea, vomiting, impetigo, scabies or lice, diaper rash, feeding problems, or failure to thrive. Additional concerns include Hepatitis B, Tuberculosis, intestinal parasites, Hepatitis C and nutritional disorders such as rickets and iron-deficiency anemia. Children may also experience transitional depression when they first meet their new parents if they have left caregivers who have developed relationships with them. Parents should be advised to tell their pediatricians that their child might likely have intestinal parasites, which are common in international adoptees, and to have them checked for their presence. The most common form of intestinal parasites is Giardia, and parents need to be alerted that worms may be passed in the stool for months to years after arrival and treatment (Aronson, 2000). Although most parasites are not transmitted from person to person, Giardia is transmitted and may result in discomfort for family members.

Parents are advised to have their child seen by their pediatrician within 10-14 days after the parents and the child have had time to recover from jet lag. Acute illness problems should be seen within 24 hours of arrival. A common error made by primary care physicians (Aronson, 2000) is to omit the recommended screening because they feel the child has been examined for a U.S. immigration visa and looks healthy.

Immunizations should be started over if records are incomplete or questionable. Medical examinations are performed by pediatricians who may then refer evaluations of sensory functions in infants, and developmental screening and assessments to occupational therapists. A partnership between a physician and an occupational therapist has been successful in some international adoption clinical programs. Usually one month is a good time for the developmental evaluation after the child has been seen by the pediatrician and has had time to settle into his/her new home life. From the author's experience, translators have only been needed for developmental assessments when an older child is adopted. Formal developmental assessments identify areas of delay and focus attention on areas for intervention and referrals. Developmental testing may introduce parents to normal sequences in development and serve as a baseline for measuring progress over time (Aronson, 2000). Children under the age of eighteen months may benefit from an evaluation of their sensory functions using assessments such as the Test of Infant Sensory Functions in Infants (DeGangi & Greenspan, 1989). Checklists of sensory difficulties can help to determine whether the child is a candidate for further Sensory Integration testing and intervention. All parents can benefit from resources on appropriate developmental and sensory motor activities for their children.

Parental interviews and clinical behavioral observations of post-institutionalized children may likely reveal problems of rocking, head banging, biting, hitting, high pain thresholds, trance-like spells, daredevil behaviors, lack of sense of safety, nightmares or night terrors (Fahlberg, 1991; Miller, 2000). Children may appear depressed and grieving for lost caregivers, and may not be comfortable with unfamiliar foods, language and new environments (Fahlberg, 1991). They may show signs of indiscriminate attachment such as overfriendliness and lack of anxiety around strangers. Post-adoption stress and fatigue may affect adoptive parents after the arrival of their child (Hopkins-Best, 1997). Empathetic listening and guidance from the occupational therapist can be an important factor for the successful transition for both parents and adoptive children.

Community Referrals, Consultations

Parents of internationally adopted children are advised to be prepared to assess and monitor their children's development on an ongoing basis and to become educated about community resources that are available for children with developmental delays. Parents can experience a great deal of satisfaction from their children as long as they can accept the fact that therapists, tutors and behavioral guidance may be necessary resources to access. Since children adopted from orphanages have typically been deprived of normal sensory input such as touch, movement, auditory and visual stimulation, sensory integration is highly regarded by adoptive parents as helpful for their children.

Early childhood stimulation programs, developmental gymnastic resources, and music groups are common referrals to help with an internationally adopted child's development. A recommendation to treat the child at the developmental level instead of the chronological age is helpful for the parent to determine what pre-school and school programs would be appropriate to consider. All children adopted from orphanages have some degree of developmental delay that should be considered when making decisions about the child's school placement. Parents may prefer to keep their internationally adopted children in younger aged classes to allow them the opportunity for additional social and school readiness performance to develop.

Support Groups, Seminars

Participation in support groups for parents and their internationally adopted children has been found helpful for families to connect with others who have experienced similar journeys. Laning (1999) works with intercountry adoptions and suggests that discussions and activities that are organized to cover the normative issues of growing up and how adoption affects these issues is helpful information for families. Often support groups are organized for a particular age such as playgroups for pre-schoolers and discussion groups for older children. Some support groups are organized by a particular ethnic heritage.

Occupational therapists can organize seminars and special discussion groups to discuss behaviors that are typical at certain developmental ages. Interactions with other internationally adopted children can help the child feel positive about being an adopted person and knowing other children in similar situations. Family pot luck dinners, camping trips, and family parties can be organized by the support group (Laning, 1999). Frequently individuals who are considering international adoption or are waiting for their child enjoy learning from the adoptive experiences of other parents and meeting their children. Some support groups take the form of grass roots organized reunions for families who have adopted from a particular country. The reunion for families who have adopted children from Romania occurs every two years in a different region of the United States. At this reunion, opportunities for seminars, play activities and lectures from health and education professionals combine with family vacations for positive experiences for the children and their parents. Occupational therapists can participate in the organization of such reunions and offer to present relevant topics to the parent groups.

CONCLUSION

As Fazio (2000) states, "there has never been a time when our return to community as our context for practice is more appropriate or more needed" (p. xi). With the increasing number of internationally adopted children in communities, the need exists for occupational therapists to expand their knowledge and practice to encompass this population. The rewards of facilitating successful adoptions for both the parents and the children are gratifying.

REFERENCES

Ames, E., Fisher, L., Morison, S. & Chisholm, K. (1999). Some recommendations of a study of Romanian orphans adopted to British Columbia. In T. Tepper, L. Hannon & D. Sandstrom (Eds.). *International adoption challenges and opportunities* (pp. 35-41). (Available from Parent Network for the Post Institutionalized Child, P.O. Box 613, Meadow Lands, PA 15347).

Aronson, J. (2000). Medical evaluation and infectious considerations on arrival. *Pediatric Annals, 29,* 218-223.

Bowlby, J. (1958). The nature of the child's tie to his mother. *International Journal of Psycho-Analysis, 39,* 350-373.

Crumpecker, L. (1997). *Health and developmental issues facing our children.* (Available from Families for Russian and Ukranian Adoption, P. O. Box 2944, Merrifield, VA 22116).

Day, S. (1982). Mother-infant activities as providers of sensory stimulation. *American Journal of Occupational Therapy, 36,* 579-585.

DeGangi, G. A. & Greenspan, S. I. (1989). *Test of sensory functions in infants (TSFI) manual.* Los Angeles: Western Psychological Services.

Faber, S. (2000). Behavioral sequelae of orphanage life. *Pediatric Annals, 29,* 242-248.

Fahlberg, V. I. (1991). *A child's journey through placement.* Indianapolis, IN: Perspective Press.

Fazio, L. S. (2000). *Developing occupation-centered programs for the community.* Upper Saddle River, NJ: Prentice Hall, Inc.

Federici, R. S. (1998). *Help for the hopeless child.* Alexandria, VA: Dr. Ronald Federici and Associates.

Haradon, G. (1999a). Sensory integration therapy and children from deprivational environments. In T. Tepper, L. Hannon & D. Sandstrom (Eds.), *International adoption: Challenges and opportunities* (pp. 87-96). (Available from Parent Network for the Post Institutionalized Child, P.O. Box 614, Meadow Lands, PA 15347).

Haradon, G. (1999b). Rehabilitation in Romania: The post-communist era. In R. Leavitt (Ed.), *Cross-cultural health care: An international perspective for rehabilitation professionals* (pp. 235-246). London: W.B. Saunders Co. Ltd.

Haradon, G., Bascom, B., Dragomir, C. & Scripcaru, V. (1994). Sensory functions of institutionalized Romanian infants: A pilot study. *Occupational Therapy International, 1,* 250-260.

Hopkins-Best, M. (1997). *Toddler adoption.* Indianapolis, IN: Perspectives Press.

Immigration and Naturalization Service: Immigrant orphans admitted to the United States by country of origin or region of birth 1989-1998. Washington, DC, Department of Justice, 1998.

Jenista, J. A. (1997). Russian children and medical records. *Adoption/Medical News, 3,* 1-8. Palm Bay, FL: Adoption Advocates, Press.

Jenista, J. A. (2000). Preadoption review of medical records. *Pediatric Annals, 29,* 212-215.

Johnson, D. (1999). Adopting an institutionalized child: What are the risks? In T. Tepper, L. Hannon & D. Sandstrom (Eds.), *International adoption: Challenges and opportunities* (pp. 8-11). (Available from Parent Network for the Post Institutionalized Child, P. O. Box 614, Meadow Lands, PA15347).

Johnson, D. E. (2000). Long-term medical issues in international adoptees. *Pediatric Annals, 29,* 234-241.

Johnson, D., & Hostetter, M. (1999). Planning for the health needs of your institutionalized child. In T. Tepper, L. Hannon & D. Sandstrom (Eds.), *International adoption: Challenges and opportunities* (pp. 12-24). (Available from Parent Network for the Post Institutionalized Child, P. O. Box 614, Meadow Lands, PA 15347).

Laning, B. (1999). Do adoptive families live happily ever after? In A. Merrill (Ed.). *Report on intercountry adoption* (p. 30). (Available from International Concerns for Children, 911 Cypress Drive, Boulder, CO 80303-2821).

Merrill, A. (Ed.). (1996). *Report on intercountry adoption.* (Available from International Concerns for Children, 911 Cypress Drive, Boulder, CO 80303-2821).

Miller, L. C. (2000). Initial assessment of growth, development, and the effects of institutionalization in internationally adopted children. *Pediatric Annals, 29,* 224-232.

Ochs, T. (2000). The internet and international adoption information. *Pediatric Annals, 29,* 249-250.

O'Connor, T. G., Rutter, M. & English & Romanian Study Team. (2000). Attachment disorder behavior following early severe deprivation: Extension and longitudinal follow-up. *J. Am. Acad. Child Adoles. Psychiatry, 39,* 703-712.

Provence, S. & Lipton, R. (1962). *Infants in institutions.* New York: International Universities Press.

Zeanah, C. H. (2000). Disturbances of attachment in young children adopted from institutions. *Developmental and Behavioral Pediatrics, 21,* 230-236.

Using Chaos Theory
to Understand a Community-Built
Occupational Therapy Practice

Sharon Elliott, OTR/L, BCN
Skip O'Neal, OTR/L
Beth P. Velde, PhD, OTR/L

SUMMARY. Community-built occupational therapy programs interact with a wide range of systems. This interaction does not occur in an orderly manner, but in an unpredictable fashion. The use of chaos theory may help program developers understand actual and potential interactions that may occur. To illustrate the use of chaos theory, a case study is presented. *[Article copies available for a fee from The Haworth Document Delivery Service: 1-800-342-9678. E-mail address: <getinfo@haworthpressinc.com> Website: <http://www.HaworthPress.com> © 2001 by The Haworth Press, Inc. All rights reserved.]*

KEYWORDS. Chaos theory, systems theory, case study, dialogal research

---

Sharon Elliott is Instructor, Pitt Community College, Occupational Therapy Assistant Program; and works at Therapeutic Innovations, Greenville, NC.

Skip O'Neal is an Occupational Therapist: I at Caswell Center, Kinston, NC.

Beth P. Velde is Associate Professor and Graduate Coordinator, Occupational Therapy Program, East Carolina University.

[Haworth co-indexing entry note]: "Using Chaos Theory to Understand a Community-Built Occupational Therapy Practice." Elliott, Sharon, Skip O'Neal, and Beth P. Velde. Co-published simultaneously in *Occupational Therapy in Health Care* (The Haworth Press, Inc.) Vol. 13, No. 3/4, 2001, pp. 101-111; and: *Community Occupational Therapy Education and Practice* (eds: Beth P. Velde, and Peggy Prince Wittman) The Haworth Press, Inc., 2001, pp. 101-111. Single or multiple copies of this article are available for a fee from The Haworth Document Delivery Service [1-800-342-9678, 9:00 a.m. - 5:00 p.m. (EST). E-mail address: getinfo@haworthpressinc.com].

Community-built occupational therapy programs must operate within complex and chaotic systems common in community settings. The purpose of this article is to describe a community-built occupational therapy program using chaos theory as a way to understand the interactions between the program and other community systems. Comprehension and use of chaos theory provides a way to plan for community-built occupational therapy programs.

METHODOLOGY

Using a case study approach, data was collected via observation, examination of artifacts and interviews. During two on-site visits two graduate students and one faculty member from East Carolina University, Department of Occupational Therapy observed and recorded data on interactions, materials and objects within the physical environment of the Northern Moore Occupational Therapy Program (NMOTP). This data included hand drawn maps of the physical space, recording of furnishings, decorations, objects, photographs of the exterior, field notes describing observed therapy sessions, and a review of the resource library. The two graduate students conducted two separate focus groups that included representatives from social services, the Northern Moore Family Service Center, parents, the contracted occupational therapists, and the staff of NMOTP. The faculty member interviewed the program coordinator on three separate occasions (twice face to face and once on the telephone). Agency documents such as brochures, policy manuals, and a review of local news articles provided additional data.

Data was analyzed collaboratively by the graduate students and the faculty member. Using the dialogal method (Halling & Leifer, 1991), preliminary dialogue explored the individual opinions of each member of the research team regarding NMOTP as a complex system. Next, common themes were mutually identified and compared to the tenets of systems theory. Finally, fundamental dialogue built on previous themes and interwove those themes to provide a consistent description of NMOTP as a complex system.

What follows is the description of the Northern Moore Occupational Program compiled from the analysis of the data through the perspective of chaos theory.

THE NORTHERN MOORE
OCCUPATIONAL THERAPY PROGRAM

The NMOTP is a unique service designed to assist families who have children ages birth through adolescence in need of occupational therapy services. The organization is a community-built occupational therapy program offering services to children with sensory integrative dysfunction. Founded in 1995 by Mary Farrell, a parent, it offers occupational therapy services for children residing in Moore and surrounding counties in this rural area of North Carolina. The program was viewed as a community-built program based on the description provided earlier in this volume (Wittman & Velde). As a community-built program, NMOTP offers skilled occupational therapy services based upon a collaborative and interactive model. The program was initiated through community efforts and the services are continually evolving based upon the community needs. While portions of the services revolve around sensory integration needs of children, the organization provides wellness programs oriented to the parents and citizens of Moore and surrounding counties.

Under the sponsorship of the Northern Moore Family Resource Center (NMFRC) and currently located in the Davis Community Center, Robbins, North Carolina, the NMOTP has been financed through fund raising events such as raffles, contributions from the United Ways of Moore and Randolph County, in-kind donations from the county commissioners, and a Kate B. Reynolds grant, which expired in 1999. The NMOTP approached the faculty at East Carolina University (ECU), Department of Occupational Therapy seeking assistance with funding limitations. One faculty and two graduate students collaborated with the organization for the purpose of increasing the funding base. Chaotic systems theory was chosen by the ECU participants as a way of understanding the complex interaction of systems and subsystems contributing to the diverse funding of this community-built organization.

As part of the NMFRC, the Northern Moore Occupational Therapy Program supports the mission of NMFRC, "to encourage the development of strong families, healthy children, and caring communities by matching resources with needs in the northern Moore County area." Through individualized occupational therapy intervention based on sensory integration theory, Parents in Action, resource and equipment lending libraries, parent workshops, special events oriented towards community education, and consultation to other human service professionals, the NMOTP offers what no other agency provides in this geographical area.

Opening in 1995 with one part-time occupational therapist (OT) treating seven children, the program currently contracts three part-time occupational therapists from an agency located approximately 70 miles away. The diagnoses of the children served at NMOTP include: attention deficit disorder with and without hyperactivity, cerebral palsy, Down's Syndrome, autism, dyspraxia, sensory defensiveness, Fragile X Syndrome, learning and behavioral problems.

Like many community-built agencies, the program continues because of a strong consumer base. Parents of children receiving occupational therapy treatment serve on standing committees, volunteer for equipment and facility maintenance, and plan for the future of the program through the Vision Task Force. Ms. Farrell continues as an integral member of the organization despite the "graduation" of her son from the program! Furthermore, the program has a significant level of endorsement from other agencies and professionals. Legislators and physicians have expressed support for the program evidenced by their letters of endorsement.

CHAOS THEORY AND NMOTP

NMOTP is a social system composed of a group or collection of entities for which there is a unifying principle. The system contains elements consisting of individuals (children and families receiving occupational therapy service), groups of individuals (such as the Advisory Committee or Vision Committee), administrative structures (such as the program coordinator, occupational therapists), and/or role sets (such as parent, client, teacher) that support the social system. For a system to exist there must be a relationship between the elements (the mission of NMOTP) and a way to distinguish the elements and their relationships from the rest of the world (membership in NMFRC and NMOTP). Systems are frequently seen as layers with one system subsumed within another. NMOTP exists within the larger layers of the

NMFRC. Boundaries between the two entities are described using administrative levels, funding sources, and client groups (see Figure 1).

CHAOS THEORY REVIEW

Chaos theory describes a system as an open entity consisting of related elements. There is a continuous flow of energy moving through the system and between the system and its environment. The system is viewed as gaining energy from its environment, creating a myriad of changes. For NMOTP this flow of energy includes the information exchanged, the flow of people in and between layers of the system and adjoining systems, and the interjection of new ideas from consultants.

The interaction of randomness, structure and time occurs within a set of rules. These rules consist of the policies and procedures of the system, the job descriptions of the people in the system, and the policies of the funding agencies. Sometimes these rules are congruent. Other times the rules contradict each other, adding new information to the system and contributing to the chaotic nature of its function.

FIGURE 1. Model of NMOTP

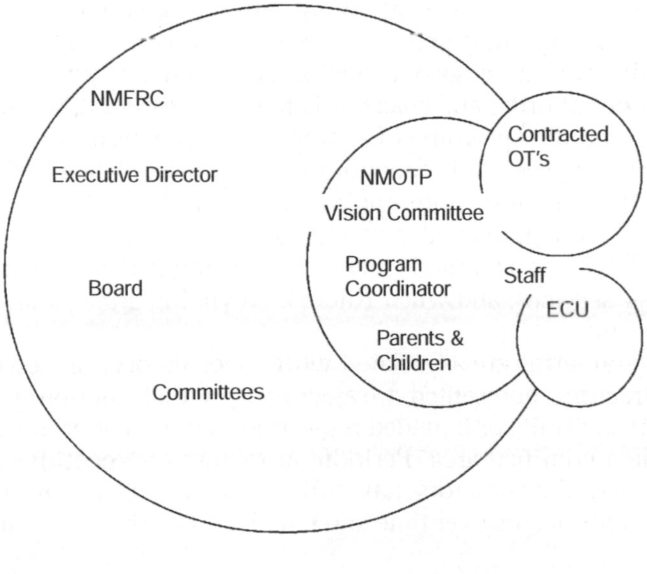

Chaos theory is a branch of mathematical science that attempts to understand the underlying order in processes that appear so complex they do not have any underlying guidelines or principles. These processes typically involve the interaction of several elements over time. The rate of change of any one element is variable and dependent upon the other elements and the interactions taking place. Predictability is difficult to achieve, not because of lack of knowledge regarding the individual elements involved, but because of the complexity of their interaction and the inaccuracy of measuring information at some arbitrary starting point in time. "Chaos demonstrates that a system can have complicated behavior that emerges as a consequence of simple, nonlinear interaction of only a few components" (Krippner, 1994, p. 53).

Bertalanffy (1969) suggests an open system

> . . . maintains itself in a continuous inflow and outflow, a building up and breaking down of its components, never being, so long as it is alive, in a state of chemical thermodynamic equilibrium but maintained in a so-called steady state which is distinct from the latter. (p. 39)

Community-built occupational therapy programs are perceived as open systems in constant interaction with their physical, natural, temporal, social and political environment. This is the primary reason chaos theory was chosen as one way to understand the NMOTP.

Transition points identifying system change are called bifurcations. These are important points in the development of the system. Phase transitions or the "edge of chaos" occur when the system is operating at the border of order and chaos. It is here, at this point, when creative activities and the spawning of entrepreneurial activities are most opportune and the system is functioning at its highest level of functioning. Examples of bifurcation points for NMOTP occurred when Ms. Farrell's son graduated and she decreased her participation in the NMOTP, when a dramatic increase occurred in the numbers of families seeking services, and when Kate B. Reynolds grant funding was in its final years.

Several terms are associated with chaos theory. In Newtonian physics attractors represented a trajectory to which motion gravitates. Attractors are finite or bounded regarding their behavior; they do not spill outside a confined area. Periodic attractors are repetitive in behavior. These periodic attractors may pull a system in chaos toward an orderly shape. This occurs over time and may be difficult to see at a single point in time. For NMOTP periodic attractors include the organization's vision, goals and strategic plan.

Chaotic or strange attractors are the "product of nonlinearity and interactivity" (Marion, 1999, p. 16). The unpredictability of strange attractors is a function of their dependence on initial conditions and the difficulty in accurately measuring these conditions at any point in time. In addition, the interaction of the attractors produces potential energy. Upon interaction, the behavior of the chaotic attractors is unpredictable. The interaction may assume a measure of synchronicity, the behavior may become dissonant, or the interaction may move the system to a transition point. Examples for NMOTP include changes in the local culture such as the increase of Hispanic residents, the introduction of new state funding such as North Carolina Health Choice, and the unexpected offers of collaboration by government officials.

Periodic attractors may provide the system with a "self-reference," allowing the system to "keep a memory of its evolutionary path" (Schalock & Bud, 1994, pp. 221-222). Strange or chaotic attractors may not be predicted nor explained in terms of causal relationships, but they can be described. However, chaotic attractors are always far from equilibrium (described in self-organization science as a state of death or non-life) (Scott, 1991).

"Dissipative system" refers to a system that, when closed, uses all its energy and fails to transform or grow. This is called "entropy" or the quantity of energy not available to a system for change. However, when a dissipative system is open, it exchanges incoming energy for entropy, keeping the system alive (Prigogine & Stengers, 1984). Open, dissipative systems actively avoid equilibrium to avoid deteriorating. This is termed negentropy. If NMOTP or its parent organization the NMFRC were to isolate themselves from their environment and discontinue their search for new members and new ideas, entropy could eliminate their ability to function. This is often seen when boards of directors' membership becomes stagnant and the organization subsequently loses its leadership and its volunteers.

OCKERMAN'S FACTORS APPLIED TO NMOTP

According to Ockerman (1997) there are five factors that determine whether a system can move into the edge of chaos (or beyond into disintegration); the rate of information flow, the degree of diversity, the richness of connectivity, the level of contained anxiety, and the degree of power differentials. These factors provide a potential tool that community-built occupational therapy programs can use for planning.

Rate of information flow. Within systems information flows in, through, and out of the system using a variety of channels. The rate of flow determines how much of the information can be acted upon and what can be attended to. Systems cognizant of the importance of information to their stability and potential growth identify the primary sources of information and provide support for the use of information. NMOTP determined three types of information as crucial at this point in their development. These included the Internet, occupational therapists, and written materials. NMOTP owns donated computers where Internet access for staff, parents and therapists enhances acquisition of up to date information on occupational therapy, sensory integration dysfunction, and learning disabilities. Use and management of the information is monitored using the program coordinator and volunteers.

The acquisition and use of a video camera and film to document the occupational therapy intervention sessions and Parents in Action meetings would allow greater access to the occupational therapists as sources. For example, parents unable to attend meetings could still benefit from the speakers by checking out a selected videotaped meeting. Videotaping intervention sessions would allow the parent(s) to use the information as a model for follow-up regarding the therapist's suggestions.

The resource and equipment library supports parents in need of written information or who wish to try out a piece of equipment before purchase. The library is utilized on a need basis by family members. An evaluation process helps to monitor the usability of the resources and to identify additional needs.

Each of these sources of information needs to be available to users in sufficient quantities and available at convenient times to meet the needs of the user. This access to information provides constituents of NMOTP the knowledge needed to promote program growth.

Degree of diversity. Complex systems involve interaction with the community outside the boundaries of the NMOTP system. This diversification beyond traditional system elements includes other agencies, families and children not currently served, and individual human service professionals. NMOTP diversifies the systems with which they interact through three types of services.

For example, the citizens residing in the counties served and human service professionals interacting with children receiving NMOTP services attend Therapy Day. This program is a special event that is focused on the community at large. Through an open house and invited speakers, attendees learn about NMOTP and sensory integrative disorders.

The educational sessions offered at Therapy Day give participants a more thorough understanding of children who have impairments in sensory integration, developmental skills, or learning. Participants acquire techniques to help the children function better in the classroom, at home and in other environments.

Second, free screening programs provided in the community help to identify children who exhibit signs of sensory integrative dysfunction and offer written resources to families regarding associated problems and potential solutions. Lastly, a newsletter is published once a month and distributed to a mailing list of approximately 1,100 individuals to apprise them of the upcoming events of both NMOTP and NMFRC, provide monthly columns written by parents and professionals, and inform the readers of other resources which meet the identified mission statement.

The NMOTP now provides assistance to a significant percentage of the Hispanic population. Over 5,440 people in the Moore County and surrounding area are of Hispanic origin (US Census Bureau, 1999). This recent demographic shift has forced NMOTP and NMFRC to provide all written information in both English and Spanish.

These intentional initiatives oriented toward diversification of the system provide the potential for strange attractors that pull the system slightly out of stability, allowing for creativity.

The richness of connectivity. Within the system, strong efforts to remain focused on a philosophy and mission allow the system some stability. Functioning as a periodic attractor, the strategic plan, organized by the Vision Committee, focuses on actualizing the philosophy of the system. In concert with direct intervention oriented toward the child, the NMOTP offers services to parents and significant others who are associated with the child. This is essential because of the disruption of relationships, diminished roles, and difficulties in educational outcomes that may be associated with sensory integrative dysfunction. Parent programs include a 12 session Parents in Action educational program. Each session lasts approximately 120 minutes and free childcare is provided to those who need it. Because parents also need social and emotional support, the NMOTP is proposing a monthly support group where, under parental leadership, parents will be offered a forum for discussing problems and engaging in problem solving strategies.

Containing the level of anxiety. Reactions to chaotic systems include the development of anxiety. The diverse and unstable funding for direct services is representative of a transition that many grass roots organizations face. Within NMOTP, many children and their families have insignificant or no financial resources to pay for such OT services. In Moore County, approximately 40% of the children below the age of five are eligible for Medicaid due to a low household income. Eighteen percent of the children in this county live below the poverty line and approximately 30% are from a single parent family (*The Pilot,* 1996). The waiting list for NMOTP services of financially needy children has been growing at a rate of 6-8 per year. This is a much higher growth rate than the current subsidies available. This has created significant anxiety since its inception for NMOTP. Its response has been to develop and expand sponsorship funding. Such funding provides children access to the occupational therapy services they require, ensures available and affordable transportation to obtain the services, and helps them access services which are located within a reasonable driving distance.

A second response to anxiety is illustrated in NMOTP's proposition to East Carolina University, Department of Occupational Therapy. Through seeking consultation with university resources, the NMOTP sought external expertise to address the instability created by insufficient funding for expansion.

Degree of power differential. The staff of an organization frequently manages the response to the effects of periodic and strange attractors and the edge of chaos. The Therapy Program Coordinator holds a 32-hour a week position. Her job description includes scheduling of all clients, maintaining appropriate supplies, maintaining files, being a contact person, giving families referral packets of information, setting up family conferences, responding to phone messages, and copying therapy information as needed. The coordinator is also responsible for arranging parent and community education programs, writing the newsletter articles, and helping with fundraising or grant writing efforts. Two therapy aides work approximately 12 hours a week and are responsible for cleaning the therapy room and equipment. They also complete tasks as assigned by the coordinator to assist in running the program. The driver or Transportation Assistant works approximately 12 hours a week and is responsible for arranging and providing transportation services for those individuals who lack transportation to obtain services at NMOTP. As a result of this myriad of responsibilities of staff, employees feel a lack of control and a lack of power to respond to the edge of chaos. Staff burnout is a significant issue that must be addressed for this system to continue to function.

Because of its grass roots origins, the NMOTP has maintained a strong volunteer core. Yet, signs of volunteer burnout have appeared. Lack of attendance at Advisory Committee meetings, a lack of clarity regarding relationships with the NMFRC Board, and the mixed roles played by the contracted occupational therapists (staff and volunteer) have further contributed to a feeling that the system is spinning in chaos.

CONCLUSIONS

The intent of this paper was to document a case study of a community-built occupational therapy program and to understand it using chaos theory. Ockerman's five factors were particularly useful in analyzing the case study data and understanding the significant strengths and weaknesses of the system in managing the edge of chaos. The analysis was a way to describe the state of the organization. One outcome of the analysis was the development of a database to be used for grant applications.

REFERENCES

Bertalanffy, L. (1969). *General systems theory.* New York: George Braziller.

Krippner, S. (1994). Humanistic psychology and chaos theory: The third revolution and the third force. *Journal of Humanistic Psychology 34* (3):53.

Marion, R. (1999). *The edge of organization: Chaos and complexity theories of formal social systems.* Thousand Oaks, CA: Sage Publications.

Ockerman, C. (1997). Facilitating and learning at the edge of chaos: Expanding the context of experiential education. 1997 AEE International Conference Proceedings. Eric reproduction services ED414123.

Prigogine, I. & Stengers, I. (1984). *Order out of chaos: Man's new dialogue with nature.* New York: Bantam Press.

Schalock, M. D. & Bud, F. (1994). The house that traces built: A conceptual model of service delivery systems and implication for change. *Journal of Special Education,* 28: 203-208.

Scott, G. P. (1991). Introduction: Self organization science and the interdisciplinary Tower of Babel syndrome. In G. P. Scott (Ed.), *Time, rhythms, and chaos in the new dialogue with nature,* pp. 3-22. Ames, IA: Iowa State University Press.

The Pilot. (1996, May 16). Author.

US Census Bureau (1999, March 22). 1990 US census data [On-line]. Available Internet: <http://www.venus.census.gov/cdrom/lookup>.

Development of a Community-Based Return to Work Program for People with AIDS

Brent H. Braveman, MEd, OTR/L

SUMMARY. This article overviews the needs assessment and program development process conducted by an occupational therapist in partnership with a community-based agency. The resulting work rehabilitation program for persons living with HIV/AIDS and based on the Model of Human Occupation is utilized as a case example to illustrate the process. The needs assessment of the target population, the processes of organizational and environmental assessment and the resulting program design and program evaluation are discussed. *[Article copies available for a fee from The Haworth Document Delivery Service: 1-800-342-9678. E-mail address: <getinfo@haworthpressinc.com> Website: <http://www.HaworthPress.com> © 2001 by The Haworth Press, Inc. All rights reserved.]*

KEYWORDS. AIDS, return to work, community-based practice

Brent H. Braveman is Clinical Assistant Professor, Department of Occupational Therapy, University of Illinois at Chicago.

Appreciation for assistance with this article and with the ongoing development of programming for people with AIDS is given to Dr. Gary Kielhofner, Karen Goldstein, and Lauren Goldbaum. A special acknowledgment is also given to Rob Humrickhouse, the Howard Brown Health Center, and the Department of Education's Rehabilitation Services Administration for their support and vision.

[Haworth co-indexing entry note]: "Development of a Community-Based Return to Work Program for People with AIDS." Braveman, Brent H. Co-published simultaneously in *Occupational Therapy in Health Care* (The Haworth Press, Inc.) Vol. 13, No. 3/4, 2001, pp.113-131; and: *Community Occupational Therapy Education and Practice* (eds: Beth P. Velde, and Peggy Prince Wittman) The Haworth Press, Inc., 2001, pp. 113-131. Single or multiple copies of this article are available for a fee from The Haworth Document Delivery Service [1-800-342-9678, 9:00 a.m. - 5:00 p.m. (EST). E-mail address: getinfo@haworthpressinc.com].

INTRODUCTION

The purpose of this article is to describe the process that was employed to partner with a community-based agency in order to develop a work rehabilitation program based on an occupational therapy conceptual practice model, the Model of Human Occupation. The intent is to provide an outline of the steps included in this process, examples of the information collected during each stage, factors that influenced decision making throughout the process, and the resulting actions that contributed to successful program development.

THE AGENCIES AND THE PROBLEM

The Howard Brown Health Center (HBHC) is a community-based organization located on the North-side of Chicago with the mission of meeting the health care needs of Chicago's Gay and Lesbian population. In the spring of 1997 staff members at HBHC identified that an increasing number of unemployed people living with AIDS were expressing interest in returning to work. Historically services provided to this population focused on maintaining quality of life while preparing for an inevitable death. People who developed symptoms secondary to AIDS were frequently counseled to leave their jobs and go on private or public disability to assure medical care during the last years of their lives. For much the same reason, persons with AIDS who were unemployed and on public assistance were not strongly encouraged to seek employment.

However, promising new pharmacological treatments had recently been introduced and had begun to give renewed hope to persons with AIDS. These treatments have since been credited with substantial decreases in HIV-related mortality since their introduction (Feinberg, 1996; Hogg, O'Shaugnessy, Gatarac, Yip, Craib, Schecter, & Mantaner, 1997). According to the Centers for Disease Control and Prevention (CDC), the number of AIDS deaths decreased in 1996 for the first time from 50,700 to 39,200 (CDC, 1997). This dramatic decrease in deaths has led to an overall increase in the number of people living with AIDS. The CDC estimated that in 1999, 412,471 persons were living with HIV/AIDS in the US (CDC, 1999). Of this number, 96% were between the ages of 19 and 64, or of prime working age.

In addition to the reduced mortality rates, the new treatments help to improve the health and function of persons living with AIDS. Consequently, many people with AIDS have experienced a return of previously lost functional capacities. Others did not experience the decline in function previously associated with AIDS. As this phenomenon evolved, clients who previously sought counseling and assistance with the process of preparing for death now began to approach the staff of HBHC for counseling and assistance with the process of living. This was illustrated by the words of one client interviewed early in the needs assessment process who summarized his feelings by saying, "It was difficult when they told me that I was going to die; but being told that I was going to live was even more difficult. What do I do now?"

In order to explore the dimensions of persons with AIDS who desired and were potentially capable of returning to work, HBHC conducted a survey in the fall of 1997 of people affected by AIDS. Fifty-five responses to the survey were collected using a convenience sample. The average respondent was 38 years old, lived alone, had at least some college level education and was last employed 3.5 years ago. Eighty-two percent of respondents had already discussed returning to work with their case manager. Two-thirds of the respondents felt optimistic about returning to work, though none of these respondents had yet returned to any form of employment.

Respondents identified a number of important barriers to re-entering the workplace. Seventy-eight percent of respondents were unsure of the impact that working might have on their health status and unsure of whether they could maintain the routine of full-time employment. Sixty-two percent of respondents were unsure of their functional capacity and its adequacy to the demands of work. Eighty percent of the respondents described the inertia secondary to a significant period of interruption of work and to prolonged illness. Because of their uncertainties, nearly 80 percent of the respondents felt they should try temporary or part-time positions before attempting to return to permanent or full time employment. Most (90%) expressed that while they had an interest in returning to work, they also had severe misgivings about the impact that returning to work might have on their ability to maintain their health benefits. Additional concerns identified included the necessity of disclosing personal information, how to address the gap in their employment history and a hesitation to ask for special consideration from employers in regard to schedules and other factors.

Concurrent with these efforts by the HBHC, the Department of Occupational Therapy at the University of Illinois at Chicago (UICOT) was recognizing a need of its own. Historically the department had relied heavily on the clinical services branch of the department located in the university medical center to provide opportunities to students for clinical observations and experiences. With changes in reimbursement that resulted in shifts in clinical practice including downsizing of staff and increased demands for productivity, it became more difficult for medical center staff to provide the same level of support to the academic unit that they had. During this same time, changes in occupational therapy practice in general were occurring. These changes included an increased focus on community-based practice (Baum & Law, 1998; Brownson, 1998; McColl, 1998). As a result of these multiple influences, it was decided that the Director of Clinical Services for the University of Illinois at Chicago Medical Center should pursue development of community-based clinical programming. This decision was made so that the range of service involvement of the academic department would more closely mirror current trends toward community-based practice being observed in occupational therapy practice as a whole. As a first effort the Medical Director of the HBHC was contacted and subsequently the Director of Special Projects was asked about the perception of the need for occupational therapy services. Discussions were begun that led to an eventual partnership focusing on meeting the needs of both agencies. These discussions occurred over a series of weeks and included specific efforts by the Director of Clinical Services to educate HBHC personnel to occupational therapy and convince them that as an occupational therapy consultant, he had something unique and important to offer. Also, the Director of Clinical Services had to learn enough about HBHC and its clients to convince other important stakeholders at HBHC that he was truly invested in the Center and its clients.

The UICOT has a considerable history in the development of work-related programming and assessments. Two other work programs have been operated by the UICOT including the Work Readiness Program for persons with mental illness and the Worksite Program for injured workers (Braveman, Sen & Kielhofner, 2000; Olson, 1998). A number of assessments have been developed and validated by the UICOT and used in these work programs, including the Worker Role Interview (WRI), the Work Environment Impact Scale (WEIS), the Occupational Self-Assessment (OSA), the Occupational Performance History Interview (OPHI-II), and the Assessment of Communication and Interaction Skills (ACIS) (Baron, Kielhofner, Goldhammer, & Wolenski, 1998; Forsyth, Salamy, Simon & Kielhofner,1998; Kielhofner, Mallinson, Crawford, Nowak, Rigby, Henry & Walens, 1998; Velozo, Kielhofner, & Fisher, 1998). Because of these assessments, the support of local experts, and the Director's established skills as a manager, the HBHC agreed to contract with the Director to develop and run a pilot vocational rehabilitation program for HBHC's clients. Howard Brown Health Center received a small grant from the National AIDS Fund in Washington, D.C., for the programming. The pilot program was well received and the HBHC and the UICOT agreed to partner to pursue permanent funding for the program. In the fall of 1998 a $729,000, three-year research and demonstration grant from the U.S. Department of Education's Rehabilitation Services Administration was acquired to develop and expand the Employment Options Program. The remainder of this article will present the process utilized in developing the program as a case history.

PROGRAM DEVELOPMENT: A CASE HISTORY

Grossman and Bortone (1986) outline an easy to follow process to guide occupational therapists with development of clinical programs. There are four steps to program development. These steps include: (1) needs assessment, (2) program planning, (3) program implementation, and (4) program evaluation. Each of these steps will be discussed using the development of the Employment Options Program as a case example.

Step One: Needs Assessment

Grossman and Bortone (1986) described a needs assessment as a process of data gathering and problem identification including a description of the target population and an assessment of the treatment needs and the resources available to meet these needs. Demographic analysis is a first step in describing the target population. Most organizations collect basic information on the individuals that they serve, including age, gender, race, employment status, educational level, and income level. In addition, it is important to identify what other information it may be necessary to obtain regarding the population. For example, the shared problems of the population in question and factors known to influence the outcome of the services must be considered as important sets of data. In the case of persons living with HIV/AIDS who desire to return to work, it was relevant to consider both health and social factors known to relate to the specific disease. These included the complexity of medication schedules, side effects of medications, and co-morbidities such as substance abuse, mental illness, or AIDS-related dementia.

Data was collected regarding factors known to influence the success of individuals attempting to return to work after disability (e.g., prior level of satisfaction with work, the individual's perception of the work environment and peer and supervisor support). To aid with program development a thorough literature review of 44 studies defining factors related to the prediction of return to work was conducted. It was subsequently published. This allowed planners to gain insight into the relationship between the symptoms and impact of AIDS on function and the process of attempting to return to work (Braveman, 1999). This review categorized the most commonly investigated factors in terms of an occupational therapy conceptual practice model, The Model of Human Occupation (Kielhofner, 1995).

While basic demographic descriptions of potential clients may be obtained by a review of existing records within the agency, other information about the particular needs and challenges of your intended population may not be readily accessible. It is easy to imagine a picture of potential clients as summary statistics such as those in Table 1 are reviewed.

However, this picture may be skewed, incomplete or missing important subtleties that are not easily shown in summary statistics. For instance, neither the demographic information available at HBHC nor the survey conducted by HBHC revealed important information about potential Employment Options clients. An example of such information was the number of clients who stated that they were unemployed but in fact were working part-time, but "under the table" in order to not jeopardize receipt of public income and insurance benefits. Acquisition of this information created a very different picture of the initial Employment Options clients. A second example of important information not readily apparent through demographic analysis was the renegotiation of roles and acceptance of additional responsibilities in the home because one life-partner (the client) was unemployed. One participant described himself as becoming the "stereotypical housewife," who, while not par-

TABLE 1. Demographics of Howard Brown Health Center Clients

Gender		Race		Age		Income	
Male:	79%	White:	52%	Under 20:	10%	<$7,741	26%
Female:	21%	Black:	29%	20-29:	28%	$7,741-$13,545	11%
		Hispanic:	12%	30-39:	25%	$13,546-$19,350	6%
		Asian:	1%	40-49:	14%	$19,351-$25,115	6%
		Unknown:	16%	50-59:	6%	$25,115-$30,960	4%
				Over 60:	2%	Over $30,960	20%
				Unknown	15%	Unknown	26%

ticipating in paid employment, managed most of the tasks related to maintaining the home. These tasks included cleaning, laundry, grocery shopping, and meal preparation. This story was repeated by a number of the initial participants and alerted staff regarding the needs of some clients to renegotiate roles in the home with their significant others. These two examples justify the use of interviews in which potential clients not only are asked about anticipated needs, but also are asked to become partners in the program design process where they are viewed as "experts" in their own lives and needs.

In the development of the Employment Options Program, narrative interviews were conducted with the 20 participants in the pilot phase of the program. The interviews included the Occupational Performance History Interview (OPHI-II) as well as targeted questions related to HIV/AIDS and return to work [e.g., How compliant are you with your medication schedule? Tell me about your understanding of your options for returning to work under the Social Security Disability Income program (Kielhofner et al., 1998)]. It is important to note that the content of the interviews did not remain static. The interviews were staggered in time so that the first three interviews were recorded and transcribed, then reviewed and analyzed for themes. New questions prompted by these themes were then incorporated into the next set of eight interviews. In turn these interviews were transcribed and analyzed to identify themes. These additional themes were used to add questions to the remaining 9 interviews. Interviews always concluded with the question, "Is there anything that I did not ask that you feel it is important for me to know in order to understand your story?" As a result the image of these clients was more complete and textured than the stark image painted by the initial demographic information available.

A third strategy employed in the needs assessment involved gathering information from organizational staff regarding their perceptions of needs of the target population. Data was gathered using key informant interviews and focus groups. At this time the possible discrepancies between what has been termed "perceived needs," "felt needs" and "real needs" was examined (Grossman & Bortone, 1986). Perceived needs are those needs identified by staff through anecdotal experience or observation that have not been validated by the target population as accurate. Felt needs are those stated by members of the target population that may not match the abilities and limitations of the target population or that would not in fact be the highest priority for clients if they truly had all the facts upon which to make an educated decision. For instance, a number of participants in the Employment Options Program pilot stated that needing help in identifying job vacancies was their most immediate need without realizing the potential negative impact on their public medical benefits. Felt needs are often supported at face value or appear congruent with demographics (e.g., assuming that groups with low education would benefit from beginning to prepare for a GED). Real needs match the true functional abilities and disabilities of the population and can be validated by objective evaluation instruments.

In the Employment Options Program design phase, key staff and key informants in the community (e.g., staff from other AIDS service organizations) were interviewed about the perceived needs of persons with HIV/AIDS who were unemployed. These perceptions were concurrently validated or rejected during the narrative interviews conducted with the pilot program participants.

Step Two: Program Planning

Grossman and Bortone (1986) suggest five elements in program planning. Each of these elements will be discussed as they were applied to the development of the Employment Options Program.

1. *Defining a focus.* Grossman and Bortone (1986) describe the key to defining a focus of a program is to identify those needs that are a priority for the majority of the target population. In the case of Employment Options it was evident that the majority of clients had four concerns: the impact of returning to work on their benefits (e.g., SSI/SSDI), disclosing their HIV status to potential employers, explaining extended gaps in their work histories and managing symptoms such as fatigue while returning to work. When the needs shared by the majority of the target population are identified, assessment of whether those needs can be met by someone else must be determined. For example, all clients of the Employment Options Program had a need for ongoing case management services, but most were already receiving these services by the Howard Brown Health Center or another AIDS service organization.

2. *Adopting a frame of reference.* Mosey (1989) described a frame of reference as the mechanism for linking theory to practice. In order to be useful for program development, a frame of reference must: (a) clearly identify its domains of concerns, (b) be based upon sound theory, (c) describe a view of the nature of occupational function and dysfunction, and (d) include technologies for application of its theory base to daily practice. In practice, therapists often draw upon multiple frames of ref-

erence to comprehensively serve their clients. For example, in the case of Employment Options, the Model of Human Occupation was chosen as the primary frame of reference because it provided a framework for understanding the individuals' occupational function and dysfunction within both the work and home environments. The Model of Human Occupation had been utilized previously both with persons with AIDS and in the study of persons with occupational dysfunction in the worker role (Azhar, 1996; Corner & Kielhofner, 1996; Corner, Kielhofner, & Lin, 1997; Mallinson, 1995; Munoz & Kielhofner, 1995; Olson, 1998; Pizzi, 1990; Velozo, Kielhofner, & Fisher, 1998). In addition to the Model of Human Occupation, other frames of reference were utilized to provide guidance for program development and intervention when the Model of Human Occupation did not provide sufficient guidance. For example, the Contemporary Task-Oriented Approach (Mathiowetz & Bass Haugen, 1994) provides specific strategies for intervening with neurological deficits not addressed in detail by the Model of Human Occupation.

3. *Establishing goals and objectives.* The next element of the program planning step is to establish goals and measurable objectives that are problem oriented and described in behavioral terms. These objectives must clearly describe what clients should be able to do once they complete the program (Grossman & Bortone, 1986). Table 2 includes sample goals and objectives developed for the Employment Options Program. Goals and objectives must be developed through a collaborative process involving all key stakeholders in the program. Included in the development of goals and objectives for Employment options were key decision-makers including the Head of the academic Department of Occupational Therapy at UIC and the Executive Director of HBHC in addition to the Director of Special Projects and the Director of Clinical Services. Clients can and should be involved in identifying and validating planned goals and objectives. To formalize this process, clients should be included on the planning committee and/or a client advisory panel.

4. *Establishing methods to integrate the program.* Inserting a new program into an existing pattern of service delivery can create numerous challenges and requires considerable forethought to avoid as many problems as possible. Grossman and Bortone (1986) suggest paying particular attention during this phase to the establishment of timelines, definition of roles, responsibilities and areas of collaboration with other staff in the environment, the identification of potential obstacles to the

TABLE 2. Sample Program Goals and Objectives

Goal 1: Clients will be educated to information regarding the impact of paid employment on public benefits	Objective 1.1: Identify persons in the community who can act as subject matter experts in SSI, SSDI and private disability insurance and the impact of paid employment on these benefits	Begin: 9/97 End: 10/97
	Objective 1.2: Develop written materials and worksheets to provide to clients with examples of how paid employment will specifically impact them	Begin: 9/97 End: 12/97
Goal 2: Clients will be able to self assess current habits and activities and the impact of introducing new occupations on their daily lives	Objective 2.1: Evaluate the NIH Activity Record as a possible assessment for use with clients	Begin: 10/97 End: 11/97
	Objective 2.2: Develop a minimum of 5 agreements with local businesses for part-time internships to allow clients to introduce work activities into their daily lives to evaluate the impact on function	Begin: 10/97 End: 4/8 with ongoing revision

implementation of the program and key resources that are necessary for success.

Because Employment Options was being developed via a collaboration between the UIC Department of Occupational Therapy and the Howard Brown Health Center, there were both advantages and disadvantages to integrating the program with existing services. The variety and depth of knowledge bases, educational backgrounds and experiences of persons available as resources at the two organizations was a particular advantage. At the same time the organizations had different short and long term goals, and used different measures of success for a program. As a result, a unique challenge resulted in order to proceed without alienating any key stakeholder. It was important that the Director of Special Projects recognize that the Department of Occupational Therapy's success would be measured in grant dollars obtained as funding for the program and in the number of research articles published based on data gathered within the program. In contrast, the Director of Clinical Services needed to recognize that the HBHC would measure the success of the program based on how quickly a quality service was provided and by the number of clients who were served effectively. The key to managing these dynamics and assuring that they remained an advantage rather than a disadvantage was open and direct communication about how to reach each organization's objectives without compromising the objectives of the other, or the program.

As a new program develops, defining roles can be a challenging process. Employment Options was not only introducing a new program into an existing service delivery structure, but in addition was introducing an entire organization to a new discipline. Few of the HBHC employees had had any prior contact with occupational therapy. Again, while inattention to this issue could have created insurmountable problems (e.g., role conflict caused by existing program staff feeling threatened), attending to the issue early and conscientiously allowed the needs of clients to be met while providing a relief for work demands to existing staff. A number of presentations and other educational efforts informed case managers about the program and the skills and proposed roles of the occupational therapist. This assured that functions were not duplicated and that relationships were established that were collaborative in nature and focused on delivering an efficient and effective service to the clients.

Other potential obstacles identified were successful integration of the program with medical services, and how other community-based AIDS service organizations in Chicago would perceive the development of this program. Both of these issues related to the perceived mission of the HBHC. Mission analysis is important in the development of any new program (Braveman, 1993). Prior to utilizing valuable resources, organizations need to ask, "Do we exist as an organization to meet these needs?" or "Is this particular service within the intended scope of what we are funded to provide?" Howard Brown Health Center's mission states:

> *The mission of Howard Brown Health Center is to promote the well-being of gay, lesbian and bisexual persons through the provision of health care and wellness programs including clinical, educational, social service and research activities.*

As plans for Employment Options proceeded, persons both internal and external to HBHC raised concerns about whether vocational rehabilitation services "fit" the mission of the organization. The medical leadership at HBHC questioned how the provision of vocational rehabilitation services fit with the mission of meeting the "healthcare" needs of Chicago's Gay and Lesbian population. In similar fashion, some staff members with other AIDS service organizations in Chicago appeared to view HBHC as primarily "medical" and perceived the development of vocational rehabilitation services as potentially encroaching on their territory. As with other obstacles, specific planned actions (e.g., meeting with medical staff individually to answer questions and offering to collaborate with other agencies) designed to allay the concerns of these stakeholders helped facilitate progress and minimize resistance.

5. *Developing referrals.* The process of developing referral systems includes three primary components: (a) evaluation protocols, (b) crite-

ria for entering and leaving each level of the program, and (c) exit or discharge criteria.

Evaluation protocols. Information from the needs assessment regarding the specific needs of persons living with AIDS and factors previously demonstrated to predict return to work after the onset of injury or disability informed the process of choosing evaluations. Use of evaluations that allowed investigation of the full range of factors shown to influence return to work after an illness or the onset of disability with each client was imperative. The primary evaluation selected was the Occupational Performance History Interview (OPHI-II). The OPHI-II is a semi-structured interview designed to provide information about the occupational performance and history of clients (Kielhofner et al., 1998). The OPHI-II allows exploration of all of the client's roles, social contacts and any of the environments in which the client operates. In addition, other evaluations were identified that could be used in conjunc-

TABLE 3. Assessments Utilized in the Employment Options Program

Assessment	Use/focus
Occupational Performance History Interview (OPHI-II) (Kielhofner et al., 1998)	Used as an initial assessment in combination with assessments of performance components. Semi-structured interview that can be administered over multiple sessions requiring 40-90 minutes depending on the client. Provides narrative information on the client's occupational performance and history including the client's roles and physical and social environments.
Occupational Self-Assessment (Baron et al., 1998)	Used as part of an initial assessment battery and as part of a goal setting process. Portions of the assessment can be conducted outside of treatment sessions after initial directions by the OT. Requires 30-60 minutes of therapist time for explanation and discussion/interpretation. Assesses the client's level of satisfaction with his/her occupational competence and environment. By examining the difference between how much a client values an item, and his/her perception of competence, a process of goal establishment for change may be incorporated.
Assessment of Communication and Interaction Skills (Forsyth et al., 1998)	Used for assessing the impact of disease/illness on communication and interaction skills. Administered through observation of a social interaction mutually agreed upon by the client and the therapist. Observation and scoring varies from 20-60 minutes. Provides scores on 20 skill verbs in three domains.
Worker Role Interview (Velozo et al., 1998)	Used for gathering information on the psychosocial/environmental components during an initial assessment process in conjunction with observations made during physical capacity evaluations or observation of performance of occupations. Semi-structured interview requiring 30-60 minutes and 10-15 minutes for scoring.
Work Environment Impact Scale (Corner et al., 1998)	Used to assess the clients' experience and perceptions of their environments. Semi-structured interview recommended for use with individuals who are currently employed or those not presently working but anticipating returning to a specific job or type of work. The interview and scoring require approximately 40-50 minutes.

tion with the OPHI-II when additional information was needed. A brief description of these assessments is included in Table 3.

Criteria for entering and leaving each level of the program. In the case of the Employment Options Program, it first seemed easy to identify criteria for entry to the program. The program was being developed for people living with AIDS who were unemployed and it seemed that these two criteria would identify who fit the program and who did not. Clients were excluded from the program if they admitted to current dependence on drugs or alcohol. Likewise, the criteria for discharge from the program was client employment.

While these criteria were accurate and are still being utilized, several surprises required evaluation of entry and discharge criteria. For example, calls were received from people who were working, but who considered themselves "underemployed." These individuals were in paid positions but may have returned to work out of necessity in an emergency situation such as to pay their rent to avoid losing their apartment. A number of these individuals had significant employment histories in professional positions such as hospital administrators or information technologists prior to their illness. While working to pay the rent and feed themselves, these individuals saw the transition back to their prior line of work as their real challenge. Depending on the specific needs of each person, (a) he or she was admitted to the program, (b) alternative individual plans of intervention were designed, or (c) referral was made to other services if a single element of assistance (such as resumé preparation) was required.

Step 3: Program Design and Implementation

During program design and implementation the Model of Human Occupation was used as an organizing frame of reference. According to the Model of Human Occupation (Kielhofner, 1995), four main factors influence work behavior. These factors are volition, habituation, performance and the environment. Volition refers to the process by which a person experiences, interprets, anticipates and chooses occupational behaviors. Habituation refers to the processes that maintain a pattern and regularity in everyday life. Performance refers to one's innate capacities that are the foundation for skilled performance. Impairments, which restrict performance, may prevent or alter how persons engage in occupational behaviors. The environment is conceived as having both a social (occupational forms and social groups) and a physical (spaces and objects) dimension. The Model emphasizes that all occupational behavior (and in this case work-behavior) is always a result of the interaction of these four elements. Ordinarily, a single factor alone does not sufficiently account for work failure or success. Consequently, the key to understanding how any person performs and experiences his or her work is to examine the intersection of that person's volition, habituation, and performance abilities with the physical and social environment.

From this view of occupational function/dysfunction, the Employment Options Program was organized in four phases and emphasizes both individual occupational therapy and group education/support sessions. In phase one, clients are assessed utilizing the Occupational Performance History Interview (OPHI-II) (Kielhofner et al., 1998). The education and support sessions are designed to help clients explore and develop both work skills and the daily habits needed to support a vocational role. Sessions include self-assessment and vocational planning, information sharing related to economics, public and private health benefits, the Americans with Disabilities Act, and job search and job skill development exercises. Phase one lasts eight weeks and is designed to provide (a) an opportunity for self-assessment and strengthening and refinement of vocational choice, (b) a structured routine to develop habits of promptness, consistency and a commitment to the program, (c) a forum for sharing critical information about returning to work, (d) a community of emotional support for return to work, (e) a context wherein factors that impact on work readiness are identified and addressed, and (f) opportunities to develop job relevant skills.

Phase two focuses on continuing to develop work skills and habits by helping clients to pursue part-time or full-time volunteer positions or internships. These experiences also allow the client to experiment with his or her tolerance for work or with management of issues such as fatigue or side effects from medication regimens. Not all clients choose to participate in phase two, and the duration and intensity of this phase is variable and is adjusted to the clients' needs. It typically varies from one to three months.

Phase three consists of placement in part-time or full-time paid employment, return to a formal educational program, or entry into a job-training program. A full-time Vocational Placement Specialist assists clients with preparation of resumes and for job interviews. At this time clients make decisions about the critical issue of disclosing their HIV status. If clients take direct advantage of opportunities developed by the program and request that an interview is arranged, disclosure of their HIV status is a foregone conclusion. Some clients perceive this as a benefit and appreciate knowing that the employer must be supportive of employing persons with AIDS by virtue of their participation with the program. Other clients prefer not to disclose their HIV status and seek employment opportunities on their own with coaching from program staff.

Phase four consists of long-term follow-up and support. Because AIDS is a chronic condition and periods of illness or functional limitation may occur, it is important that program staff is available to intervene and provide support as needed. Clients take considerable periods of time to adjust to new and more complicated role repertoires that come with returning to work. In addition, clients who may encounter difficulties after months of successful employment not anticipated when first returning to work. For example, clients may not perceive the need to make requests for reasonable accommodations under the Americans with Disabilities Act may later find this process necessary as they manage side effects such as fatigue or diarrhea accompanying changes in medications.

Table 4 illustrates the assessments used in the program and sample intervention strategies that correlate with each of the subsystems of the model.

Step 4: Program Evaluation

The aim of program evaluation is to measure the effects of a program compared to the goals it is designed to accomplish in order to improve the program (Grossman & Bortone, 1986). Program evaluation guides the decision making process by providing data that will help determine if programs should continue, be discontinued or changed.

Program evaluation can include both formal and informal strategies to collect and analyze the data that will guide decisions about how to improve the program. Formal methods, such as tracking client outcomes, assisted in measuring the effectiveness of the Employment Options Program. Outcomes tracked to evaluate program success included the number of clients who were enrolled in the program versus those who completed each phase of the program or withdrew from the program. Examples of other formal outcome measures include the number of clients placed in internships, or the number of clients who entered paid employment, formal education or job training programs. In addition, in the case of Employment Options there were outcomes considered as indicators of success by occupational therapists that did not match the initial goal of the program. One example would be a client

TABLE 4. Employment Options Program Elements and the Model of Human Occupation

Model of Human Occupation	Assessments Utilized	Sample Intervention Strategies

Volitional Subsystem
  Values
  Interests
  Personal Causation
    Knowledge of Capacity
    Sense of Efficacy
	Occupational Performance
	  History Interview
	Occupational Self-Assessment
		Volunteer experiences to develop and explore new interests and test capacity for work
		
		Group education/support sessions to explore values and desires regarding work and tangible and intangible benefits/rewards of working

Habituation Subsystem
  Roles
  Habits
	Worker Role Interview
	NIH Activity Record
	Role Checklist
		Examination of how work will impact current occupations and re-negotiating roles in the home with significant others
		
		Use of leisure activities in the community to increase activity and develop habits and skills such as punctuality and time management skills

Mind-Brain-Body Performance Subsystem	Assessment of Motor
	  and Process Skills
	Assessment of Communication
	  and Interaction Skills
		Attendance at computer lab sessions to develop work skills
		
		Internships in local businesses to build skills and improve capacities for work

Environment(s)
  Home
  Former Work Settings
  Anticipated Work Settings
	Work Environment Impact Scale	Attendance at local job fairs to practice socialization in a work/business environment

who must face the difficult decision that returning to paid work is not a realistic option. If in the process of the program the client is able to incorporate other occupations into his or her life and expresses increased satisfaction with their life despite remaining unemployed, this would also denote a "successful" outcome. Through the process of ongoing program evaluation, changes and improvements are constantly being made to the Employment Options Program to deliver more effective intervention for the clients.

INITIAL PROGRAM OUTCOMES

Eighty-six clients have enrolled in the Employment Options Program since receiving federal funding from the U.S. Department of Education's Rehabilitation Services Administration. Of this number, 26 (30%) have failed to complete the program. Clients who failed to complete the program were often also struggling with the complication of substance abuse or mental illness in addition to AIDS.

Of the 60 clients who have completed the program, 32 (37%) have returned to paid employment or are currently involved in a formal educational program to prepare them for a new career. Twenty-eight clients (33%) are in the early phases of the program and are participating actively in internships or skill development efforts with program staff. While it is early to fully evaluate results of the program, these initial results are promising. In addition, program staff are currently collaborating with two supported living residences for people with AIDS in Chicago. This effort is focused on increasing involvement of persons with multiple diagnoses (for example, AIDS and substance abuse) who have a lower rate of completing the program.

CONCLUSION

Program development can be a daunting process further complicated when conducted in a community-based setting unfamiliar with occupational therapy. However, the use of a working model such as that presented by Grossman and Bortone (1986) and descriptions of actual program development such as the one presented here can make this task easier. Further expansion of services into the community and to evolving populations of persons with disabilities such as AIDS can bring great rewards for both the profession of occupational therapy and individual practitioners. A program development model such as that illustrated in this article can be used as a tool to foster success.

REFERENCES

Azhar, F.T. (1996). *The relevance of worker identity to return to work in clients treated for work related injuries.* Unpublished Masters Thesis, University of Illinois at Chicago, Chicago, Illinois.

Baron, K., Kielhofner, G., Goldhammer, V. & Wolenski, J. (1998). *A user's manual for the OSA: The Occupational Self-Assessment.* Chicago, IL: Department of Occupational Therapy, University of Illinois at Chicago.

Baum, C., & Law, M. (1998). Nationally speaking–community health: A responsibility, an opportunity, and a fit for occupational therapy. *American Journal of Occupational Therapy, 52,* 7-10.

Braveman, B.H. (1993). The basics of marketing occupational therapy services. In *Promoting the profession: A resource guide for marketing and publicizing occupational therapy.* Bethesda, MD: The American Occupational Therapy Association.

Braveman, B.H. (1999). The model of human occupation and prediction of return to work: A review of related empirical research. *Work: A Journal of Prevention, Assessment & Rehabilitation, 12*, 13-23.

Braveman, B.H., Sen, S., & Kielhofner, G. (2000). Community-based vocational rehabilitation programs. In M. Scaffa (Ed.), *Occupational therapy in community-based practice settings.* Philadelphia, PA: FA Davis.

Brownson, C.A. (1998). Funding community practice: Stage 1. *American Journal of Occupational Therapy, 52*, 60-64.

Centers for Disease Control and Prevention. (1997). *HIV/AIDS surveillance report, 9*, No. 1. Atlanta, GA.

Centers for Disease Control and Prevention. (1999). *HIV/AIDS surveillance report, 11*, No. 2 Atlanta, GA.

Corner, R. & Kielhofner, G. (1996). The Work Environment Impact Scale. Chicago, IL: Department of Occupational Therapy, University of Illinois at Chicago.

Corner, R., Kielhofner, G., & Lin, F.L. (1997). Construct validity of a work environment impact scale. *Work, 9*, 21-34.

Feinberg, M.B. (1996). Changing the natural history of HIV disease. *Lancet, 348*, 239-246.

Forsyth, K., Salamy, M., Simon, S., & Kielhofner, G. (1998). *A user's guide to the assessment of communication and interaction skills (ACIS) Version 4.0.* Chicago, IL: Department of Occupational Therapy, University of Illinois at Chicago.

Grossman, J., & Bortone, J. (1986). Program development. In S.C. Robertson (Ed.), *Strategies, concepts, and opportunities for program development and evaluation.* (pp. 91-99). Bethesda, MD: The American Occupational Therapy Association.

Hogg, R.S., O'Shaugnessy, M.V., Gatarac, N., Yip, B., Craib, K., Schecter, M.T., & Mantaner, J.S. (1997). Decline in deaths from new antiretrovirals (letter), *Lancet, 349*, 1294.

Kielhofner, G. (1995). *A model of human occupation: Theory and application* (2nd Edition). Baltimore, MD: Williams & Wilkins.

Kielfhofner, G., Mallinson, T., Crawford, C., Nowak, M., Rigby, M., Henry A., & Walens, D. (1998). *A user's manual for the occupational performance history interview.* Chicago, IL: The Model of Human Occupation Clearinghouse, University of Illinois at Chicago.

Mallinson, T. (1995). Work Programs at Hinsdale Hospital: Addressing Work in Mental Health Settings. Chicago, IL: Department of Occupational Therapy, University of Illinois at Chicago.

Mathiowetz, V., & Bass Haugen, J. (1994). Motor behavior research: Implications for therapeutic approaches to central nervous system dysfunction. *American Journal of Occupational Therapy, 48*, 733-745.

McColl, M.A. (1998). What do we need to know to practice occupational therapy in the community. *American Journal of Occupational Therapy, 52*, 11-18.

Mosey, A.C. (1989). The proper focus of scientific inquiry in occupational therapy. Frames of reference (Editorial). *Occupational Therapy Journal of Research, 9*, 195-201.

Munoz, J.P., & Kielhofner, G. (1995). Program development. In G. Kielhofner (Ed.), *A Model of Human Occupation: Theory and application* (2nd ed.) Baltimore, MD: Williams & Wilkins.

Olson, L. (1998). *Work readiness: Day treatment for persons with chronic disabilities.* Chicago, IL: Model of Human Occupation Clearinghouse, Department of Occupational Therapy, University of Illinois at Chicago.

Pizzi, M.A. (1990). The model of human occupation and adults with HIV infection and AIDS. *American Journal of Occupational Therapy, 44,* 257-264.

Velozo, C., Kielhofner, G., & Fisher, G. (1998). A user's guide to the worker role interview (Version 9). Chicago, IL: Department of Occupational Therapy, University of Illinois at Chicago.

Development of Occupational Therapy in a Homeless Shelter

Georgiana Herzberg, PhD, OTR/L
Marcia Finlayson, PhD, OT (C), OTR/L

SUMMARY. This paper describes a program which provides occupational therapy services to a population of homeless individuals residing in an emergency shelter in Ft. Lauderdale, Florida. Principles of community-built practice were combined with the use of the Canadian Model of Occupational Performance to provide the theoretical approach for the program. A needs assessment was done and the programming developed and implemented based on identified needs is described. Outcomes and recommendations for the future are discussed. *[Article copies available for a fee from The Haworth Document Delivery Service: 1-800-342-9678. E-mail address: <getinfo@haworthpressinc.com> Website: <http://www.HaworthPress.com> © 2001 by The Haworth Press, Inc. All rights reserved.]*

KEYWORDS. Homeless populations, community building, program development

Georgiana Herzberg is Associate Professor of Occupational Therapy, Nova Southeastern University, 3200 S. University Drive, Ft. Lauderdale, FL 33328. Marcia Finlayson is Assistant Professor of Occupational Therapy, University of Illinois at Chicago [MC811], 1919 West Taylor Street, Chicago, IL 60612.

The authors wish to thank NSU doctoral students Amy Russell, OTR/L; Tina Gelpi, OTR/L; and Elisa Honeyman, OTR/L; and TSA staff Marta Munoz, MSW, Warren Smith, and Harold Dom, MSW, for their work in making this program a success.

[Haworth co-indexing entry note]: "Development of Occupational Therapy in a Homeless Shelter." Herzberg, Georgiana, and Marcia Finlayson. Co-published simultaneously in *Occupational Therapy in Health Care* (The Haworth Press, Inc.) Vol. 13, No. 3/4, 2001, pp.133-147; and: *Community Occupational Therapy Education and Practice* (eds: Beth P. Velde, and Peggy Prince Wittman) The Haworth Press, Inc., 2001, pp. 133-147. Single or multiple copies of this article are available for a fee from The Haworth Document Delivery Service [1-800-342-9678, 9:00 a.m. - 5:00 p.m. (EST). E-mail address: getinfo@haworthpressinc.com].

Over the past decade, many changes have occurred in the everyday practice of occupational therapists. These changes have been influenced by many factors, both internal and external to the profession. Internally, there has been a reorientation to occupation and occupation-based practice (Christiansen & Baum, 1997; Moyers, 1999), as well as theoretical developments (Kielhofner, 1997; Townsend, 1997; Wilcock, 1998; Zemke & Clark, 1996), and a growing focus on health promotion and community practice (Finlayson & Edwards, 1997; Letts, Fraser, Finlayson & Walls, 1993). Externally, there have been dramatic shifts in the structure of the health, social and educational systems particularly with respect to reimbursement options and insurance caps for therapy services (Christiansen & Baum, 1997; Bailey, 1998). These changes have encouraged occupational therapists to consider the application of their skills and knowledge beyond the traditional health care system. The purpose of this article is to describe the development of occupational therapy services in a homeless shelter. This was a collaborative venture between Nova Southeastern University (NSU) and The Salvation Army of Broward County. The description of the collaboration is divided into rationale, process, and structure.

THE CONTEXT OF HOMELESSNESS IN THE UNITED STATES

According to the National Coalition for the Homeless (1999), approximately 700,000 people are homeless in the United States on any given night. The problem of homelessness in the United States, particularly within urban communities, has been the subject of increasing public attention since the early 1980s. Historically, the majority of people who were homeless were young or middle-aged men, but this fact is rapidly changing. Changes in the socioeconomic and demographic composition of the population who are homeless include an increased number of visible individuals, more families, more working poor, and an increased number of individuals suffering from problems of chronic mental illness and chemical dependency (U.S. Department of Labor, 1997). The proportions of women, children and families among the homeless population are steadily increasing and the U.S. Conference of Mayors' survey of homelessness in 30 cities found that children under the age of 18 accounted for 25% of the urban homeless population (U.S. Conference of Mayors, 1998).

Extreme poverty is felt to be the major cause of homelessness by many scholars, policy makers and lay people. Despite recent increases in the minimum wage, the real value of the minimum wage in 1997 was 18.1% less than in 1979 (Mishel, Bernstein, & Schmitt, 1999). A host of other factors also seem to have exacerbated the problem of homelessness. These include increases in restrictions on eligibility requirements for welfare and disability benefits; reductions in the purchasing power of public benefits; shortages of low-income housing; changes in deinstitutionalization policies and a lack of community services for mentally ill persons; increases in the numbers of women and children who are victims of domestic violence; and increases in the number of people experiencing problems of substance abuse (U.S. Department of Labor, 1997; Toro & Warren, 1999; Applewaite, 1997; Boyt, 1999). Extended periods of unemployment, or alternatively, employment in menial jobs with low wages, have been found to increase the risk of becoming homeless (Applewaite, 1997). As a result of these diverse issues, people who are homeless have a broad range of practical needs including finding a job, finding affordable housing, learning how to manage money, learning how to get along better with other people, handling legal issues, and utilizing resources (Applewaite, 1997; Herman, Struening & Barrow, 1994; Moxley & Freddolino, 1991).

For many individuals who are homeless, mental illness, substance abuse, and insensitive service providers complicate meeting these needs. An estimated 15% to 30% of people who are homeless have a serious mental disorder and as many as 70% of them also struggle with substance abuse/dependence (Toro et al., 1997). People who are homeless report barriers to service use such as insensitive service providers (e.g., lack of respect, worker's negative attitudes), negative policies and procedures (e.g., age discrimination, dehumanizing rules and regulations), and problems with inaccessibility, inadequate services and a generally discouraging social services system (Applewaite, 1997).

The needs of persons who are homeless also change with the length of time the individual has been homeless. Belcher, Scholler-Jaquish, and Drummond (1991) have identified three stages of homelessness: marginal, recent, and chronic. People who are considered to be marginally homeless often live close to the poverty line, and frequently use services in the community such as clothing drops and soup kitchens. Individuals who are recently homeless do not necessarily consider themselves homeless, and have many needs. They need to gain control over their lives, including assistance with locating and utilizing resources, and rebuilding social networks (Belcher et al., 1991). Health care problems increase for these individuals the longer that they stay homeless. Individuals who are chronically homeless accept their lifestyles as the norm. These individuals rarely seek services in the community; instead, street outreach workers often approach them with assistance.

RATIONALE FOR OCCUPATIONAL THERAPY IN A HOMELESS SHELTER

The Department of Labor recommends that both assessment and case management should be ongoing activities for people who are homeless because barriers to employment are not always evident at the time of intake (U.S. Department of Labor, 1997). Occupational therapists are well prepared to provide these assessment and case management services. The needs, issues and barriers facing people who are homeless are closely aligned with the skills and knowledge of occupational therapists (Heubner & Tryssenaar, 1996; Tryssenaar, Jones, & Lee, 1999) and there is a growing recognition of this alignment (e.g., Bunch, 1999; Falk-Kessler, O'Halloran & Reid, 1999; Shordike, 1999). This alignment becomes apparent when one considers the skills and philosophical basis of occupational therapy. Occupational therapy practice emphasizes the importance of client-centered engagement in meaningful and purposeful occupations. Occupational therapists also acknowledge the importance of a spiritual core (Christiansen, 1997; Townsend, 1997) and work with people to minimize the residual effects of substance abuse, mental illness, domestic violence, low self-esteem and feelings of inadequacy. Activity analysis and adaptation can be used to develop and tailor interventions to empower, remediate, and/or accommodate occupational dysfunction that may result from a life on the streets. We have the theory base, knowledge, and skills to provide meaningful interventions that facilitate occupational performance among people who are homeless.

ASSESSING THE POTENTIAL FOR OCCUPATIONAL THERAPY SERVICES

Local Context of Homelessness

The Annual Report on Homeless Conditions in Florida (1998) found over 55,000 homeless people living within the state. Sixty-eight percent of Florida's homeless population is considered new homeless while people described as chronic and long-term homeless make up the remaining 32% of the total population. It is estimated that 37% of the people who are homeless have physical disabilities and that health care problems will increase for these individuals the longer that they stay homeless (Annual Report on Homeless Conditions in Florida, 1998). As previously identified, individuals who are recently homeless do not necessarily consider themselves homeless and have many needs. They need to gain control over their lives, including assistance with locating and utilizing resources, and rebuilding social networks.

The Salvation Army (TSA) of Broward Country Shelter is a 164-bed facility housing men, women, and children in one of two programs. The short-term program of the Emergency Shelter is to help stabilize people who are homeless. The Transitional Program provides an extended time and training that is structured to prepare residents for self-sufficiency (The Salvation Army, 2000).

Defining the Clients and Negotiating the Services

This entire program collaboration was initiated with the Director of Social Services of The Salvation Army of Broward County Emergency Shelter, Ft. Lauderdale, Florida, in the spring of 1998. The needs, concerns, roles, and responsibilities of the partners (i.e., NSU and TSA) were negotiated over the course of the next six months through a series of meetings and discussions. The outcome of these negotiations was a contract between Nova Southeastern University and the shelter to provide 10 hours per week of occupational therapy services. These services are provided by a licensed occupational therapist who acts as a teaching assistant (TA) for the occupational therapy program at this site while providing services.

Once the contract was in place, more specific attention was directed to clearly defining the activities of the occupational therapist. It became apparent that there were three stakeholder groups with both complimentary and competing demands. These stakeholder groups are the people who live in the shelter, the staff of TSA, and the NSU Occupational Therapy Program. Residents had need for direct services to improve occupational performances, the primarily non-professional staff had educational needs such as ways to facilitate helping relationships and set realistic goals with residents, and NSU had needs for additional occupational therapy community placements where classroom knowledge and techniques could be applied and role modeled for students.

A major constraint to meeting these needs was the availability of members of the stakeholder groups to participate in occupational therapy programming. Before the initiation of occupational therapy services, there was no structured programming in the evenings for clients, nor was there any structured continuing education for staff. Students were accustomed to working regular daytime hours, not evening schedules at a site located in a marginalized area of Ft. Lauderdale. As a result, establishing an occupational therapy program within the context of the existing routine of the shelter was challenging. The specific challenges are described below.

Program Development Challenges

Staff members at the shelter have different levels of education, ranging from high school completion to graduate degrees. Some of the staff have been homeless themselves. Their typical workday involves doing intakes, doing information gathering and referral, and generally managing casework. Their daily routines have little free time, and any routine that exists is always subject to having to cope with a resident's crisis. Even advanced scheduling of continuing education programs does not guarantee that staff members can attend.

Residents at the shelter are a diverse group of individuals including single men and women, couples, and families with children. Approximately 10% of the shelter residents are considered medically fragile because of physical disability or chronic illness (e.g., diabetes, respiratory disease). Residents of the shelter are admitted to the shelter at 5:00 p.m. each evening, provided dinner between 5:30 and 6:30 p.m., and have lights out at 10:00 p.m. All residents except those who are medically fragile are required to leave the shelter after breakfast and by 7:00 a.m. each day. Families must be out of the shelter by 8:00 a.m. Medically fragile residents are the only ones who are allowed to remain in the shelter during the day. Consequently programming for the majority of the residents had to be scheduled between dinner and lights out. Programming for adults had to account for the potential need for childcare, as children cannot be left unattended at the shelter, or in the care of another resident.

Selecting a Guiding Theoretical Framework

From the beginning, the Nova Southeastern University team wanted to ensure that occupational therapy services were responsive to the needs of the people at the shelter and services were guided and developed with the input and assistance of the people living at the shelter. Therefore, community building (Minkler, 1997) was combined with the use of the Canadian Model of Occupational Performance (Townsend, 1997) to provide a theoretical approach to guide this project.

Community building emphasizes collaboration between service providers and services recipients, and focuses on problem resolution using strengths-based assessments and interventions. Community-built practice is the delivery of skilled services by practitioner(s) using a collaborative and interactive model with clients. It emphasizes the strengths of the client and is wellness oriented. Typically, such a practice eliminates or resolves client issues by providing expert knowledge that is not otherwise available to the client, is issue based, and ends when the client-defined community has effectively built the capacity for empowerment. Community-built practice is *not* the same as community-based practice. Community-*based* practice is skilled services delivered by a health practitioner(s) using an interactive model with clients. This model emphasizes the strengths of a specific profession in eliminating or remediating the problems of the client. Community-*based* practice is typically medical system initiated, relies on referrals from other professionals, and is on-going over time.

By focusing on strengths with a community-*built* model, the NSU team enables the people living in The Salvation Army emergency shelter to build future capacities rather than simply resolving immediate and existing problems. Using this approach has the potential to contribute to resolving problems such as insensitive service providers, negative policies and procedures, and problems with inaccessibility to health care. Applying the community building framework to the development and operation of this program means that occupational therapy does not provide solutions but *works with* the staff and clients of The Salvation Army to determine *their strengths* for building client-centered, meaningful and goal directed interventions. By applying the community-building framework, the NSU occupational therapy team minimized the use of the expert model and emphasized a model of empowerment.

We then chose to use the Canadian Model of Occupational Performance (CMOP) as our occupational therapy theoretical base (Townsend, 1997). The CMOP was chosen because of its emphasis on client-centered occupational performances, the dynamic relationship between the person, the environment, and her/his occupation, and the fact that it identifies spirituality as the core of the person with performance components (physical, cognitive, affective) surrounding it. We felt that these aspects of the model allowed us a better theoretical match between the skills and knowledge of occupational therapy, the needs of people who are homeless, and the basic principles governing interventions initiated by The Salvation Army. By combining community building theory and occupational therapy theory, the NSU team became a more effective resource for sharing skills and information previously unavailable to the persons living at the shelter and to the persons who staffed it. The mission of our collaboration with TSA is to build communities to improve the quality of life of people affected by homelessness. We will accomplish this mission through strong leadership and teamwork in occupational therapy service, education, and research. We will empower individuals and organizations in ways that will end the cycle of homelessness.

Services Implemented

Within these constraints, challenges, and our chosen theoretical framework, we began to assemble a program by conducting a needs assessment to ensure a client-centered perspective. The needs assessment involved periods of participant observation and focus groups with people living at the emergency shelter and with the people who staffed it to determine their interests, needs, and strengths. After completing the needs assessment, interventions that were developed to increase occupational performance of people living at the shelter were:

- prevocational skills to build attitudes and skills required for workforce entry/re-entry
- stress management (e.g., productive leisure skills, time management, and coping skills)
- self-care training (e.g., parenting groups, job grooming and dressing)
- social and interpersonal skills (e.g., assertiveness, self-expression, conflict resolution, basic conversational skills, and interpersonal interactions)
- community living skills training (e.g., money management, shopping, public transportation, and community resources)

The occupational therapy team's contribution was to analyze the activities in which residents participated/intended to participate and to help residents and staff identify key components necessary for success in performance so meaningful programs could be developed. In keeping with the CMOP, residents confirmed and prioritized their occupational performance needs. To help residents practice the skills needed to gain control over their lives, empowerment opportunities were embedded in our occupational therapy groups by including clients in decision-making and leadership roles.

An important vehicle for client decision-making has been the Client Advisory Board (CAB), a monthly meeting where people who are residing at the shelter have an opportunity to raise and discuss issues that are important to them with representatives of the occupational therapy team and shelter staff. Residents at the shelter have seen their concerns translated into changes to shelter policy (e.g., extension in the hours that case managers are available) and in learning opportunities focused on improving occupational performance. General themes of needs have emerged. These include the need for:

- flexibility in program times and locations so that as many people as possible can benefit from the services offered
- specialized groups for subpopulations (e.g., women, children and people who use substances)
- specific self-care skill groups (e.g., managing stress, managing interpersonal conflicts, accessing community supports and services, and developing time management skills to form more positive habits)
- specific work related skill groups (e.g., managing money, job search and application/interview skills)

While the group topics are similar to the topics we anticipated as relevant to this population, the groups are scheduled on the basis of interest as determined in the CAB meetings. Groups coordinated by the occupational therapist but organized and implemented by others include Adult Basic Education, computer skills training, faith-based interventions, substance abuse groups, and Emotions Anonymous.

The occupational therapy team has at various times offered continuing education sessions for TSA staff. Topics included mental illness, interpersonal interactions, collaborative goal setting, and goal writing. Sessions on conducting groups have been requested.

For NSU as a client of our program, the need for a site where theory and practice can come together for the Master's degree level occupational therapy students has also created demands and presented opportunities for us. Occupational therapy students have become involved in this program on a number of levels: as master's degree occupational therapy student volunteers, as students on the three week Level I fieldwork rotations for the mental health theory and practice class, and as students on Level II fieldwork. Student volunteers are required to make a commitment of six consecutive weeks to build continuity and trust with the residents. Students who have volunteered typically request a fieldwork placement at the shelter, and fieldwork students, who have not volunteered before the placement, often continue their investment after the placement is over.

Students at all of these levels have provided an important source of manpower for groups and for resource development. For example, when residents identified a need for specific information to access social services (i.e., to secure immunizations mandated for school placement of their children), students created maps to sites, collected schedules, and rode buses to determine any additional cues that could empower residents by making the trip less overwhelming. When residents identified the problem of competing for employment while using a TSA address, students organized a job fair in which employers came to the shelter on a designated evening to recruit employees.

By examining the occupational performances demands put on each of our three stakeholder groups, we have been able to construct a program that benefits shelter residents, benefits staff, and provides a unique learning opportunity for our master's level occupational therapy students. Between April 1998 and November 2000, we have had 13 Level I students, one Level II student, 20 master's level occupational therapy student volunteers, two PhD students, and two PhD volunteers.

Students typically remark on positive changes in their attitudes towards people who are homeless. One student wrote, "This experience has provided me new insights to replace old stereotypes of homeless individuals. Our clients at TSA are articulate, intelligent, and motivated people. They are appreciative of our services. I have found that OT services are both needed and wanted. As a student, it [the experience] has provided me with practical knowledge in running groups and learning how to start a new program. This experience has been very valuable to me." Another student wrote, "Through my participation in the collaboration, I have learned a great deal about community building, including how to identify stakeholders and recognizing the various levels of clients in any community or large scale setting. I have developed skills in assessing client needs and giving up the expert role along with realizing there are several levels of empowerment. I have also gained respect for the shelter residents and many of their insights into their life circumstances, their motivation to make changes and break the cycle of homelessness and problem solving abilities. I have also gained respect for the NSU and TSA teams, working with limited resources and still creating a program that helps address the client's needs."

We encourage our students to share these perspectives and we have been able to mentor our master's level occupational therapy and doctoral students in group and independent presentations about their experiences and our research at state, regional, and national conferences. We have also been able to include TSA staff in a state conference presentation.

OUR OUTCOMES

This collaboration has had an impact on residents at the shelter, TSA staff, and NSU faculty and students. The impact of this program has been positive for all stakeholder groups. From our initial collaboration with TSA in mid-1998, we have seen TSA hire a full-time occupational therapist on their staff, continue the 10 hour/week contract for occupational therapy with NSU, establish meaningful educational experiences for master's level occupational therapy and doctoral student education and research, add occupational therapy to the list of services described in their brochure, and be asked to present this program at a regional meeting of The Salvation Army providers. We have seen changes in the physical environment at the shelter resulting from our program: A lounge was converted to a classroom, a suggestion box was built by the residents and is prominently displayed and used, a storage area was converted to a computer room, resource files were created and placed in clearly identified areas, and an outside smoking area turned into a patio with native plants.

Attitudinally, we have helped to change the "homeless hotel" image described by one staff member to that of a dynamic place to get yourself together. Skills are built in the kitchen internship program initiated by a Level I occupational therapy student and conducted by the TSA chef. Skills are built in the Client Advisory Board meetings, the job skills groups on applications and interviews, and the communications skills and anger management groups.

Staff skills have been upgraded in training sessions and 1:1 interactions. Measurable outcomes and interventions are discussed. The university gets calls to expand the program to other sites, such as community mental health agencies and community feeding programs for people who are homeless.

Students see the shelter as place of hope where they can both learn and apply knowledge. All stakeholders–TSA residents, TSA staff, NSU students, and NSU faculty–are pleased with the progress we have made in the 18 months this program has been in actual operation. We have all won through this collaboration.

RECENT PROGRAM DEVELOPMENTS

While we are pleased with our accomplishments, there remains much to be done. The social ills that contribute to homelessness do not go away. For many of our residents, participation in prevocational skills development and help in securing employment do not translate into the ability to sustain meaningful, gainful employment. We believe more people-power is needed to provide the personalized, in-depth interventions often required for success with this population. We have also realized that the work skills of some residents are compromised by hearing and vision deficits.

In working to solve these two issues, we initiated a grant with the U.S. Department of Health and Human Services. In July 2000, the Health Resources and Services Administration (HRSA) funded a three-year, occupational therapy grant creating an interdisciplinary student training program at the shelter. The grant brings students and faculty from the NSU School of Optometry, the Communication Disorders Program that includes both speech-language pathology and audiology, and Dispute Resolution to work with the existing occupational therapy program in addressing work and productivity issues with the residents at TSA. We believe the residents will greatly benefit from the vision and hearing screenings and the opportunity for in-depth learning in how to manage anger and mediate conflicts. More personnel to provide an increased variety of programs allows the occupational therapy program to focus on building prevocational skills of attendance, participation, problem solving, work quantity and work quality using both group and 1:1 sessions. Specific skills of job search, resume writing, job-related grooming and hygiene, interviewing, and time management will be continued and the additional people-power afforded us by the training grant will allow more individualized attention to specific resident needs. Activities of daily living groups such as money management and budgeting will continue. The groups emphasizing awareness of community leisure and educational resources with support for resident participation in these activities will be expanded.

CONCLUSION

In summary, this paper provides an overview of the literature on homelessness in the United States and discusses how occupational therapists could provide meaningful interventions with this population. We then provide a description of the specific context for the occupational therapy interventions that we implemented in Florida, including the importance of theory in guiding all of our interventions. We document representative personal outcomes of residents of the shelter, the impact of occupational therapy at the agency level, and the expansion of the project through a federal training grant initiated and directed by the NSU Occupational Therapy Program. The grant has brought additional services to the residents of the homeless shelter with the addition of students from disciplines that have a clear relationship to increased productivity on the job. The addition of these disciplines builds upon and exponentially increases the impact our occupational therapy services. Occupational therapy services at The Salvation Army Emergency Shelter are highly valued by the residents, by the agency, and by Nova Southeastern University as a student training site that exemplifies its mission of service to the local community.

REFERENCES

Annual report on homeless conditions in Florida. (1998). Tallahassee, FL: State of Florida.

Applewhite, S. (1997). Homeless veterans: Perspectives on social services use. *Social Work, 42* (1), 19-30.

Bailey, D. M. (1998). Legislative and reimbursement influences on occupational therapy: Changing opportunities. In M.E. Neistadt & E.B. Crepeau (Eds.) *Willard & Spackman's occupational therapy* (9th ed., pp. 763-790). Philadelphia: Lippincott.

Baum, C. & Christiansen, C. (1997). The occupational therapy context: Philosophy-principles-practice. In C. Christianson & C. Baum (Eds.) *Occupational therapy: Enabling function and well-being* (2nd ed., pp. 26-45). Thorofare, NJ: Slack.

Belcher, J. R., Scholler-Jaquish, A., & Drummond, M. (1991). Three stages of homelessness: A conceptual model for social workers in health care. *Health and Social Work, 16* (2), 87-93.

Bunch, S. J. (1999, April 18). Homeless adults, life skills, and occupational therapy: What's the connection? Presentation at the AOTA Annual Conference & Exposition, Indianapolis, Indiana.

Christiansen, C. (1997). Acknowledging a spiritual dimension in occupational therapy practice. *American Journal of Occupational Therapy, 51,* 169-172.

Christiansen, C. & Baum, C. (1997). Understanding occupation: Definitions and concepts. In C. Christianson & C. Baum (Eds.) *Occupational therapy enabling function and well-being* (2nd ed., pp. 26-45). Thorofare, NJ: Slack.

Falk-Kessler, J., O'Halloran, D., & Reid, L. (1999, April 18). The relationship of living skills and cognition in individuals who are homeless. Presentation at the AOTA Annual Conference & Exposition, Indianapolis, Indiana.

Finlayson, M., & Edwards, J. (1997). Evolving health environments and occupational therapy: Definitions, descriptions and opportunities. *The British Journal of Occupational Therapy, 60,* 456-459.

Herman, D. B., Struening, E. L., & Barrow, S. M. (1994). Self-reported needs for help among homeless men and women. *Evaluation and Program Planning, 17,* 249-256.

Heubner, J. E., & Tryssenaar, J. (1996). Development of an occupational therapy practice prespective in a homeless shelter: A fieldwork experience. *Canadian Journal of Occupational Therapy, 63* (1), 24-32.

Kielhofner, G. (1997). *Conceptual foundations of occupational therapy, 2nd ed.* Philadelphia, PA: F.A. Davis Company.

Law, M., Cooper, B. A., Strong, S., Steward, D., Rigby, R., & Letts, L. (1997). Theoretical contexts for the practice of occupational therapy. In C. Christiansen & C. Baum, *Occupational Therapy: Enabling function and well-being* (2nd ed., pp. 73-102). Thorofare, NJ: Slack Incorporated.

Letts, L., Fraser, B., Finlayson, M., & Walls, J. (1993). *For the health of it! Occupational therapy within a health promotion framework.* Toronto: CAOT Publications ACE.

Minkler, M. (Ed.) (1997). *Community organizing and community building for health.* New Brunswick, NJ: Rutgers University Press.

Mishel, L., Bernstein, J., & Schmitt, J. (1999). *The state of working America: 1998-99.* Washington, DC: Economic Policy Institute.

Moxley, D. P. & Freddolino, P. P. (1991). Needs of homeless people coping with psychiatric problems: Findings from an innovative advocacy project. *Health and Social Work, 16* (1), 19-26.

Moyers, P. A. (Ed.) (1999). The guide to occupational therapy practice. Special issue. *American Journal of Occupational Therapy, 53* (3).

National Coalition for the Homeless. (1999). Who is homeless? *NCH Fact Sheet #3.* [on-line]. Available from: http://nch.ari.net/who.html.

Shordike, A. (1999, April 19). Community-based fieldwork in a homeless shelter. Presentation at the AOTA Annual Conference & Exposition, Indianapolis, Indiana.

Surber, R. W., Dwyer, E., Ryan, K. J., Goldfinger, S. M., & Kelly, J. T. (1988). Medical and psychiatric needs of the homeless–A preliminary response. *Social Work, 33* (2), 116-119.

The Salvation Army of Broward County, Ft. Lauderdale, FL. Social Services Program brochure 2000.

Toro, P., Rabideau, J., Bellavia, C., Daeschler, C., Wall, D., Thomas, D., & Smith, S. (1997). Evaluating an intervention for homeless persons: Results of a field experiment. *Journal of Counseling and Clinical Psychology, 65* (3), 476-484.

Toro, P., & Warren, M. (1999). Homelessness in the United States: Policy considerations. *Journal of Community Psychology, 27* (2), 119-136.

Townsend, Elizabeth (Ed.) (1997). *Enabling occupation: An occupational therapy perspective.* Ottawa: CAOT Publications ACE.

Tryssenaar, J., Jones, E. J., & Lee, D. (1999). Occupational performance needs of a shelter population. *Canadian Journal of Occupational Therapy, 66* (4), 188-195.

U.S. Department of Housing and Urban Development. *Review of Stewart B. McKinney Homeless Programs Administered by HUD: Report to Congress,* 1995. Available, free, from HUD User, P.O. Box 6091, Rockville, MD 20849; 1-800-245-2691.

U.S. Department of Labor: Http://www.doleta.gov/homelessness/.

Wilcock, A. (1998). *Occupational perspective of health.* Thorofare, NJ: Slack.

Zemke, R., & Clark, F. (1996). *Occupational science: An evolving discipline.* Philadelphia, PA: F.A. Davis.

Quality of Life Issues in Community Occupational Therapy Practice

Beth P. Velde, PhD, OTR/L

SUMMARY. Quality of life has long been purported to be an outcome of occupational therapy practice. Yet little outcome data is available illustrating the effectiveness of occupational therapy in enhancing quality of life. Recent authors have addressed health related quality of life issues. Community practice would also benefit from attention to global quality of life concepts and outcome measures. This article discusses global quality of life and reviews related outcome measures. *[Article copies available for a fee from The Haworth Document Delivery Service: 1-800-342-9678. E-mail address: <getinfo@haworthpressinc.com> Website: <http://www.HaworthPress.com> © 2001 by The Haworth Press, Inc. All rights reserved.]*

KEYWORDS. Objectivity, subjectivity, outcome measures, global quality of life

As early as the 1950s, quality of life as it pertains to populations was discussed in the literature, especially regarding environmental pollution and the deterioration of urban living environments (Szalai, 1980). Theorists in the 1960s began discussing quality of life from an individual

Beth P. Velde is Graduate Coordinator and Associate Professor, Department of Occupational Therapy, East Carolina University. Address correspondence to: Department of Occupational Therapy, East Carolina University, 306 Belk, Greenville, NC 27858.

[Haworth co-indexing entry note]: "Quality of Life Issues in Community Occupational Therapy Practice." Velde, Beth P. Co-published simultaneously in *Occupational Therapy in Health Care* (The Haworth Press, Inc.) Vol. 13, No. 3/4, 2001, pp. 149-155; and: *Community Occupational Therapy Education and Practice* (eds: Beth P. Velde, and Peggy Prince Wittman) The Haworth Press, Inc., 2001, pp. 149-155. Single or multiple copies of this article are available for a fee from The Haworth Document Delivery Service [1-800-342-9678, 9:00 a.m. - 5:00 p.m. (EST). E-mail address: getinfo@haworthpressinc.com].

perspective. The 1980s brought the discussion of quality of life to the field of disability, especially those with an intellectual impairment (Brown, Bayer & MacFarlane, 1989; Cummins, 1991).

The rehabilitation literature contains over 100 definitions and models of quality of life. Some apply to the general population and others are disability specific. Most authors agree that quality of life is a multidimensional construct and assume there is variability between individuals. Because an individual's lifespan is dynamic, quality of life is dynamic.

Researchers agree that quality of life must be viewed holistically, taking into account all aspects of the individual's life. These aspects are commonly grouped into domains. The domains included as part of the quality of life construct vary between authors. In addition, quality of life is viewed in three ways–as a global construct, as health related, and using a utility approach. While the utility approach using such indicators as the Gross National Product is seldom used in occupational therapy, health related quality of life models are discussed by Edwards (1997) in *Occupational Therapy: Enabling Function and Well-Being.* Global quality of life measures offer therapists in community practice the potential to address both health related factors such as physical, functional, emotional and mental well being, along with non-health related elements such as jobs, family, friends, and other life circumstances (Gill & Feinstein, 1994, p. 619).

GLOBAL MODELS OF QUALITY OF LIFE

Global quality of life models attempt to use both an objective and subjective perspective of life domains. Objective domains of quality of life may include social indicators such as income, employment, education, physical function, housing and purity of air (Stormberg, 1988). They can be assessed without consulting the individual. Because of this objective stance, these may not take into account actual individual daily experiences. As a result, a subjective stance, asking the individual his/her perspective about the life domains, allows access to the person's daily experience. As a result, many authors (Felce & Perry, 1997; Brown, Bayer, & MacFarlane, 1989; Quality of Life Research Project, 2000; Zhan, 1992) support a combined model, where both objective and subjective assessment are incorporated.

Subjective assessment includes the extent to which an individual's needs are being met relative to the objective indicators, the importance of each indicator to the individual, and his/her global perception of life satisfaction.

The interpretation of one's quality of life includes:

1. the discrepancy between a person's achieved and unmet needs and desires.
2. the extent to which an individual increasingly controls aspects of his/her life.
3. the discrepancy between the individual and the norms of one's culture regarding the objective indicators (Brown, Bayer & MacFarlane, 1989).

Perhaps the most difficult aspect of assessing an individual's quality of life arises when there is discrepancy between the objective indicators and the person's perceptions of those indicators. For example, in comparing the social indicators to others within the individual's culture, it may be evident to the practitioner that the person lives in an environment of poor quality or is receiving inadequate health care. Yet, the individual may evaluate those indicators as satisfactory. When this occurs, it is important to determine if the person is aware that better quality is possible. According to the Centre for Health Promotion (2000), individuals may believe that "they have to suppress the importance of some possibilities because of their present circumstances." This is particularly evident when individuals feel they have no power to change current circumstances.

The indicators chosen as domains within conceptual models of quality of life vary from author to author. Felce and Perry (1997) evaluated fifteen conceptual papers from writing concerned with the general population and populations of persons with a disability. From these, they concluded the domains most represented included physical, material, social, emotional and productive life domains. What is important to the practitioner in choosing a conceptual model and compatible assessment tool is to insure both are congruent with the type of occupational therapy the practitioner is employing in the community.

DETERMINATION OF QOL

Describing the construct of quality of life and choosing appropriate assessment tools based on that description is an essential step in using quality of life as an outcome measure. Gill and Feinstein (1994) clearly articulate the dilemma inherent in this process. In a review of a Quality of Life Bibliography (listing 579 articles), they found that less than half of the articles cited "quality of life" as a key term. Randomly choosing and examining 75 of the articles for face validity, they identified only 11 articles that conceptually defined quality of life and identified the domains being measured. In addition, only 13 of the 75 investigators asked for the individual's perceptions regarding his/her quality of life. This is problematic, as assessment of quality of life requires an in-depth knowledge of the person, an understanding of her/his circumstances, and insight into how s/he experiences circumstances.

After analyzing the literature on quality of life assessment, this author identified four that provide a conceptual model and are congruent with community practice in occupational therapy. The criteria used in this review included: (1) the article must have a conceptual description of quality of life, (2) the article must include a description of the domains included in quality of life, (3) the assessment must have subjective and objective measurement capabilities, (4) the assessment must have the potential to gather data from participants relative to the level of importance of each domain, and (5) the model and assessment must be congruent with occupational therapy principles.

THE QUALITY OF LIFE PROFILE

The Centre for Health Promotion (Quality of Life Research Centre, 2000) at the University of Toronto has developed a conceptual model of quality of life and nine instruments for assessment. Based on "the degree to which a person enjoys the important possibilities of his or her life," the model reflects the interaction of personal and environmental factors. The framework includes three life domains, each of which has three subdomains. *Being* includes physical being, psychological being, and spiritual being. *Belonging* includes connections with one's environments through physical, social and community belonging. *Becoming* incorporates achieving personal goals, hopes and aspirations through practical, leisure and growth becoming.

The *Quality of Life Profile: A Generic Measure of Health and Well-Being* is one example of the assessment tools available from the center. The *Quality of Life Profile* arose from the analysis of the literature on quality of life and qualitative data collected in a series of focus groups and in-depth interviews. It consists of 54 items, with six in each of the nine sub-domains. The respondent provides scores of importance and enjoyment using a five-point Likert scale. Enjoyment is operationalized on the assessment as satisfaction. A profile is created for each individual based on domain and sub domain scores.

THE QUALITY OF LIFE SCALE

Burckhardt (Burckhardt, Clark & Bennett, 1993) modified Flanagan's (1978, 1982) Quality of Life Scale by adding a 16th item, "Independence, doing for yourself." The 16 items are rated by the respondent using a seven-point Likert style scale with one being terrible and seven being delighted or pleased. The items describe a number of occupations including those related to learning, work, creativity, active recreation, socializing, volunteering and relationships. In addition, the individual rates self-understanding, health, and material comforts. Scores are summed to constitute a total score. This score can be compared to other scores that have been published using the scale.

THE QUALITY OF LIFE INDEX

The *Quality of Life Index* consists of two sections (Ferrans & Powers, 1985). The first requires the respondent to rate satisfaction and the second importance for each of 34 life domain items. Using a six-point Likert type scale the index addresses health, health care, pain, energy, independence, family and significant others, stress, environment, faith, appearance, control over life, sex life, employment, and peace of mind.

QUALITY OF LIFE QUESTIONNAIRE

Ventegodt, Hilden and Zachau-Christiansen (1999) continue to develop a variety of questionnaires and interview assessment tools based on a meta-theory of quality of life. The theoretical basis for the assessment tool incorporates the following concepts: immediate self-experience being, satisfaction, happiness, fulfillment of needs, experience of objective temporal domains-work-family-leisure, experience of objective spatial domains, expression of life's potential, and affective factors.

Each assessment developed must achieve seven goals–maintain congruence with a definition for quality of life, maintain congruence with a philosophy of human life, operationalize this philosophy of human life, provide quantifiable response alternatives, maintain adequate reliability, achieve validation through meaningfulness to researchers and respondents, and demonstrate aesthetic appeal. While the most frequently used assessment contains 317 items, the Quality of Life Research Center (2000) continues refining and designing additional assessment tools.

USE OF A MODEL
OF OCCUPATIONAL THERAPY MODEL OF PRACTICE

In an upcoming book, Velde and Fidler will discuss a phenomenologically based quality of life assessment congruent with the Life-style Performance Model. Using the four domains of the model, the assessment will ask respondents to provide occupations within each domain that contribute to their quality of life. The respondent will then rate each based upon current level of satisfaction and importance using a Likert type scale. In a second section, the social, cultural, temporal, natural, man-made, and economic environment will be treated in a similar fashion.

CONCLUSION

Occupational therapists who practice in community-based and community-built environments must be innovators and leaders in the use of quality of life as an outcome measure. Participation in occupational therapy programs offered to all citizens has the potential to enhance both the lives of individuals and the life of the community. But it is not enough to claim this outcome. It is time we support the claim through assessments compatible with occupational therapy principles.

REFERENCES

Brown, R. I., Bayer, M. B. & MacFarlane, C. (1989). *Rehabilitation programmes: Performance and quality of life of adults with developmental handicaps.* Toronto: Lugus Productions Inc.

Burckhardt, C. S., Clark, S. R., & Bennett, R. M. (1993). Fibromyalgia and quality of life: A comparative analysis. *Journal of Rheumatology, 20,* 475-479.

Centre for Health Promotion. (2000). http://www.utoronto.ca/qol/concepts.htm.

Cummins, R. A. (1991). The comprehensive quality of life scale-intellectual disability: An instrument under development. *Australian and New Zealand Journal of Developmental Disabilities, 17,* 259-264.

Edwards, D. F. (1997). The effect of occupational therapy on function and well-being. In C. Christiansen & C. Baum (Eds.), *Occupational therapy: Enabling function and well-being* (Second Ed.) (pp. 556-576). Thorofare, NJ: Slack Inc.

Felce, D. & Perry, J. (1997). In R. I. Brown (Ed.), *Quality of life for people with disabilities* (Second Ed.) (pp. 49-62). London: Stanley Thornes.

Ferrans, C. & Powers, M. (1985). Quality of Life Index: Development and psychometric properties. *Advances in Nursing Science, 8,* 15-24.

Flanagan, J. C. (1978). A research approach to improving our quality of life. *American Psychologist, 33,* 138-147.

Flanagan, J. C. (1982). Measurement of quality of life: Current state of the art. *Archives of Physical Medicine and Rehabilitation, 63,* 56-59.

Gill, T. M. & Feinstein, A. R. (1994). A critical appraisal of the quality of Quality-of-Life measurements. *JAMA, 272,* 619-626.

Quality of Life Research Center. (2000). http://home2.inet.tele.dk/fclk/index.htm.

Quality of Life Research Project. (2000). http://www.utoronto.ca/qol.

Stormberg, M. F. (1988). *Instruments for clinical nursing research.* Norwalk, CT: Appleton and Lange.

Szalai, R. (1980). The meaning of comparative research on the quality of life. In R. Szalai (Ed.) *The quality of life.* London: Sage.

Tate, D. G., Dijkers, M. & Johnson-Greene, L. (1996). Outcome measures in quality of life. *Topics in Stroke Rehabilitation, 2*(4), 1-17.

Ventegodt, S. Hilden, J., & Zachau-Christiansen, B. (visited 3/29/99). Measuring the quality of life: A methodological framework. http://home2.inet.tele.dk/fclk/mq12.htm.

Zhan, L. (1992). Quality of life: Conceptual and measurement issues. *Journal of Advanced Nursing, 17,* 795-800.

Index

T - #0570 - 101024 - C0 - 212/152/9 - PB - 9780789014061 - Gloss Lamination